Histological Typing of Tumours of the Exocrine Pancreas

Springer
Berlin
Heidelberg
New York
Barcelona
Budapest
Hong Kong
London
Milan
Paris
Santa Clara
Singapore
Tokyo

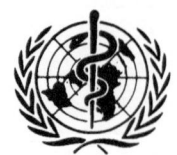 # World Health Organization

The series *International Histological Classification of Tumours* consists of the following volumes. Each of these volumes – apart from volumes 1 and 2, which have already been revised – will appear in a revised edition within the next few years. Volumes of the current editions can be ordered through WHO, Distribution and Sales, Avenue Appia, CH-1211 Geneva 27.

A coded compendium of the International Histological Classification of Tumours (1978).

The following volumes have already appeared in a revised second edition with Springer-Verlag:

Histological Typing of Tumours of the Exocrine Pancreas

G. Klöppel, E. Solcia, D.S. Longnecker,
C. Capella, and L.H. Sobin

In Collaboration with Pathologists in 7 Countries

Second Edition – Corrected Printing

With 60 Colour Figures

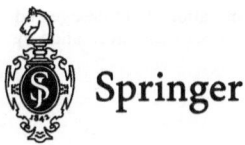 Springer

G. Klöppel
Professor of Pathology and Chairman
Dept. of Pathology, University of Kiel
Michaelisstr. 11, 24105 Kiel, Germany

D. S. Longnecker
Professor of Pathology
Dept. of Pathology
Dartmouth Medical School
Hanover, NH 03756, USA

E. Solcia
Professor of Pathology and Chairman
Dept. of Pathology, University of Pavia
Via Forlanini 14–18, 27100 Pavia, Italy

C. Capella
Professor of Pathology and Chairman
Dept. of Pathology
University of Pavia at Varese
Viale Borri 57, 21100 Varese, Italy

L. H. Sobin
Chief, Gastrointestinal Pathology
Dept. of Hepatic and Gastrointestinal Pathology
Head, WHO Collaborating Center for the Intl. Histological Classification of
Tumours, Armed Forces Institute of Pathology Washington, DC 20306, USA

First edition published by WHO in 1978 in the International Histological Classification
of Tumours series

2nd Edition 1996
Corrected Printing 1998

ISBN-13: 978-3-540-60280-4   e-ISBN-13: 978-3-642-61024-0
DOI: 10.1007/978-3-642-61024-0

CIP data applied for
Die Deutsche Bibliothek – CIP Einheitsaufnahme. International histological classification of tu-
mours/World Health Organization. – Berlin; Heidelberg; New York; London; Paris; Tokyo; Hong
Kong; Barcelona; Budapest: Springer. NE: World Health Organization
Histological typing of tumours of the exocrine pancreas/[World Health Organization]. G. Klöppel ...
In collab. with pathologists in 7 countries. – 2. ed. – Berlin; Heidelberg; New York; London; Paris;
Tokyo; Hong Kong; Barcelona; Budapest: Springer, 1996
(International histological classification of tumours)
    ISBN 3-540-60280-1
NE: Klöppel. Günter: World Health Organization
Histological typing of tumours of the exocrine pancreas. – 2. ed. – 1996

The use of general descriptive names, registered names, trademarks, etc. in this publication does not
imply, even in the absence of a specific statement, that such names are exempt from the relevant pro-
tective laws and regulations and therefore free for general use.

Product liability: The publisher cannot guarantee the accuracy of any information about dosage and
application contained in this book. In every individual case the user must check such information by
consulting the relevant literature.

Typesetting: Best-set Typesetter Ltd., Hong Kong

SPIN: 1067 1984   81/3135 – 5 4 3 2 1 0 – Printed on acid-free paper

Participants

Bogomoletz, Wladimir, Dr.
Laboratoire d'Anatomie Pathologique, Institut Jean-Godinot,
Reims Cedex, France

Capella, Carlo, Dr.
Department of Pathology, University of Pavia at Varese,
Varese, Italy

Heitz, Philipp U., Dr.
Department of Pathology, University of Zürich, Zürich,
Switzerland

Kato, Yo, Dr.
Department of Pathology, Cancer Institute, Tokyo, Japan

Klöppel, Günter, Dr.
Institute of Pathology, University of Kiel, Kiel,
Germany

Lemoine, Nicholas R., Dr.
ICRF Oncology Group, RPMS, Hammersmith Hospital,
London, United Kingdom

Longnecker, Daniel S., Dr.
Department of Pathology, Dartmouth Medical School,
Hanover, NH, USA

Morohoshi, Toshio, Dr.
First Department of Pathology, Showa University School
of Medicine, Tokyo, Japan

Pour, Parviz, Dr.
The Eppley Institute, University of Nebraska Medical Center,
Omaha, NE, USA

Solcia, Enrico, Dr.
Department of Pathology, University of Pavia, Pavia, Italy

Sobin, Leslie H., Dr.
Department of Hepatic and Gastrointestinal Pathology,
WHO Collaborating Center for the International Histological
Classification of Tumours, Armed Forces Institute
of Pathology, Washington, DC, USA

General Preface to the Series

Among the prerequisites for comparative studies of cancer are international agreement on histological criteria for the definition and classification of cancer types and a standardized nomenclature. An internationally agreed classification of tumours, acceptable alike to physicians, surgeons, radiologists, pathologists and statisticians, would enable cancer workers in all parts of the world to compare their findings and would facilitate collaboration among them.

In a report published in 1952,[1] a subcommittee of the World Health Organization (WHO) Expert Committee on Health Statistics discussed the general principles that should govern the statistical classification of tumours and agreed that, to ensure the necessary flexibility and ease of coding, three separate classifications were needed according to (1) anatomical site, (2) histological type and (3) degree of malignancy. A classification according to anatomical site is available in the International Classification of Diseases.[2]

In 1956, the WHO Executive Board passed a resolution[3] requesting the Director-General to explore the possibility that WHO might organize centres in various parts of the world and arrange for the collection of human tissues and their histological classification. The main purpose of such centres would be to develop histological definitions of cancer types and to facilitate the wide adoption of a uniform nomenclature. The resolution was endorsed by the Tenth World Health Assembly in May 1957.[4]

---

[1] WHO (1952) WHO Technical Report Series. No 53, 1952, p. 45
[2] WHO (1977) Manual of the international statistical classification of diseases, injuries, and causes of death. 1975 version. Geneva
[3] WHO (1956) WHO Official Records. No 68, p. 14 (resolution EB 17.R40)
[4] WHO (1957) WHO Official Records. No 79, p. 467 (resolution WHA 10.18)

Since 1958, WHO has established a number of centres concerned with this subject. The result of this endeavour is the International Histological Classification of Tumours, a multi-volume series whose first edition was published between 1967 and 1981. The present revised second edition aims to update the classification, reflecting progress in diagnosis and the relevance of tumour types to clinical and epidemiological features.

Preface to Histological Typing of Pancreatic Exocrine Tumours, Second Edition

The first edition of *Histological Typing of Tumours of the Liver, Biliary Tract and Pancreas* was published in 1978.[1] The WHO Collaborating Centre for that classification had been established in 1972 at the Department of Pathology, University of Hong Kong, Queen Mary Hospital Compound, Hong Kong, under the directorship of Professor J.B. Gibson. Several years ago, when the revision was planned, it was felt that each organ merited separate classification. The second edition of *Histological Typing of Tumours of the Gallbladder and Extrahepatic Bile Ducts* was published in 1990.[2] In 1994 the second edition of *Histological Typing of Tumours of the Liver* followed.[3]

This revised classification of tumours of the exocrine pancreas is based on a draft which was circulated to the participants listed on pages V and VI. After changes were made, based on their responses, a second draft was circulated and the final version elaborated. The histological classification listed on pages 11–12 contains the morphology codes of the International Classification of Diseases for Oncology (ICD-O)[4] and the Systematized Nomenclature of Medicine (SNOMED).[5]

---

[1] Gibson JB, Sobin LH (1978) Histological Typing of Tumours of the Liver, Biliary Tract and Pancreas. Geneva, World Health Organization (International Histological Classification of Tumours, No. 20)

[2] Albores-Saavedra J, Henson DE, Sobin LH (1990) Histological Typing of Tumours of the Gallbladder and Extrahepatic Bile Ducts, Second Edition. Berlin, Springer-Verlag

[3] Ishak KG, Anthony PP, Sobin LH (1994) Histological Typing of Tumours of the Liver, Second Edition. Berlin, Springer-Verlag

[4] World Health Organization (1990) International Classification of Diseases for Oncology. Geneva

[5] College of American Pathologists (1982) Systematized Nomenclature of Medicine. Chicago

It will, of course, be appreciated that the classification of tumours of the exocrine pancreas reflects the present state of knowledge, and that modifications are almost certain to be needed as experience accumulates. Nevertheless, it is hoped that, in the interests of international cooperation, all pathologists will use the classification as put forward.

The publications in the series "International Histological Classification of Tumours" are not intended to serve as textbooks, but rather to promote the adoption of a uniform terminology that will facilitate communication among cancer workers. For this reason, literature references have intentionally been omitted and readers should refer to standard works for bibliographies.

Contents

Introduction

This is a histological classification of tumours and tumour-like lesions of the exocrine pancreas which also includes those tumours showing a mixture of exocrine and endocrine elements. The classification is based principally on standard microscopic observations, but whenever indicated it incorporates diagnostically valuable immunohistological findings. In addition, the most important immunohistological findings which are helpful in categorizing pancreatic tumours are summarised in Table 1.

The major guideline of this classification scheme is the grouping of the pancreatic exocrine tumours according to their biological behaviour. Thus, the neoplasms are broadly divided into benign (adenoma) and malignant tumours (carcinoma). However, in recent years we have learned that this division is not a sharp but rather a gradual transition. We therefore added a third group which we call "tumours of uncertain malignant potential" representing a borderline category analogous to that recognized for some ovarian tumours. This group includes mucinous cystic tumour, intraductal papillary-mucinous tumour and solid-pseudopapillary tumour. These neoplasms are defined by the grade of dysplasia and/or potential to become malignant. Mucinous cystic tumours of uncertain malignant potential, for instance, exhibit moderate epithelial dysplasia, but do not show severe dysplasia/carcinoma in situ changes, nor carcinomatous invasion of the cyst wall or the adjacent pancreatic tissue. Solid-pseudopapillary tumour has a benign looking histological appearance, but metastases may occur. Biologically, all these neoplasms are primarily slow-growing lesions and have an excellent prognosis when adequately treated by complete resection. However, some of these tumours, if they are inadequately treated or remain untreated, may become frankly malignant and evolve into metastasizing carcinomas. As this behaviour may be difficult or even impossible to predict in individual tumors on the

Table 1. Differential immunohistology of epithelial pancreatic tumours

Tumour type	CK8, 18	CK7, 19	CEA	M$_1$	TRYP	NSE[d]	SYN[d]	CG[d]	AAT	VIM
Serous cystadenoma	+	+	–	–	–	–	–	–	–	–
Ductal adenocarcinoma	+	+	+	+	–	–	–	–	–	–
Mucinous cystic tumour	+	+	+	+	–	–	–	–	–	–
Intraductal papillary-mucinous tumour	+	+	+	+	–	–	–	–	–	–
Acinar cell carcinoma	+	+[b]	–	–	+	–	–	–	–[a]	–
Pancreatoblastoma	+	+	–	–/+	+	–	–	–	–	–
Solid-pseudopapillary tumour	–[a]	–[a]	–	–	–	+	–	–	+	+
Endocrine tumour	+	+[c]	–	–	–	+	+	+	–	–

CK, cytokeratin; CEA, carcinoembryonic antigen; M$_1$, peptide core antigen of mucin in gastric superficial foveolar cells; TRYP, trypsinogen; NSE, neuron-specific enolase; SYN, synaptophysin; CG, chromogranin A; AAT, alpha-1-antitrypsin; VIM, vimentin.
[a] Usually negative.
[b] Negative in about 20%–30% of cases.
[c] Negative in most cases for CK7.
[d] Focal positivity possible in ductal adenocarcinoma, mucinous cystic tumour, intraductal papillary-mucinous tumour, acinar cell carcinoma and pancreatoblastoma (see "Explanatory Notes").

basis of the currently available morphological and biological features, we believe it is appropriate to categorize them as tumours of uncertain behaviour or borderline malignant potential.

Many of the terms which are currently in use to designate the various pancreatic tumours have been retained. However, we have also introduced some new terms in the hope that these names more adequately describe the main features of the respective tumours and may be less easily confused with designations of other tumours. The most important new names are the *intraductal papillary-mucinous tumour*[1] which should replace such terms as "mucin-producing tumour" or "mucinous ductal ectasia", and the *solid-pseudopapillary tumour* which, in histological terms, is more accurate than "solid and papillary epithelial neoplasm", "solid and cystic tumour" or "papillary-cystic tumour". The term tumour is used synonymously with *neoplasm*.

---

[1] Sessa F, Solcia E, Capella C, Bonato M, Scarpa A, Zamboni G, Pellegata NS, Ranzani N, Rickaert F, Klöppel G (1994) Intraductal papillary-mucinous tumours represent a distinct group of pancreatic neoplasms: an investigation of tumour cell differentiation and K-ras, p53 and c-erbB-2 abnormalities in 26 patients. Virchows Arch 425:357–367

Table 2. Histological grading of pancreatic ductal adenocarcinoma[1]

Tumour[a] grade	Glandular differentiation	Mucin production	Mitoses (per 10 HPF)	Nuclear atypia
1	Well-differentiated duct-like glands	Intensive	≤5	Little polymorphism, polar arrangement
2	Moderately differentiated duct-like and tubular glands	Irregular	6–10	Moderate polymorphism
3	Poorly differentiated glands, mucoepidermoid and pleomorphic structures	Abortive	>10	Marked polymorphism and increased nuclear size

HPF, high power fields
[1] Klöppel G, Lingenthal G, von Bülow M, Kern HF (1985) Histological and fine structural features of pancreatic ductal adenocarcinomas in relation to growth and prognosis: studies in xenografted tumours and clinicopathological correlation in a series of 75 cases. Histopathology 9:841–856.
[a] In this system, the entire neoplasm is classified by the highest grade of any of its components, regardless of their prevalence.

Although the classification of exocrine tumours of the pancreas lists a number of different neoplasms, by far the most frequent tumour is the ductal adenocarcinoma. It accounts for 80%–85% of the cases and, together with its variants (i.e. mucinous noncystic carcinoma, signet-ring cell carcinoma, adenosquamous carcinoma and undifferentiated carcinoma), it comprises more than 90% of all pancreatic tumours. This is the reason that all incidence figures, histological grading systems and tumour stage categorizations refer to the ductal adenocarcinoma.

The incidence of pancreatic ductal adenocarcinoma in developed countries ranges between 8.0 and 12.0/100000 for males and between 4.5 and 7.0/100000 for females. Incidence rates from most developing countries range between 1.0 and 2.5/100000. Incidence and mortality rates are almost identical, since survival rates for pancreatic carcinoma are extremely low (mean 5-year survival rate 3%). Ductal adenocarcinoma has its peak

Table 3. TNM Classification of carcinomas of the exocrine pancreas (1997)[#]

Primary Tumour (T)
TX   Primary tumour cannot be assessed
T0   No evidence of primary tumour
Tis   Carcinoma in situ
T1   Tumour limited to the pancreas, 2 cm or less in greatest dimension
T2   Tumour limited to the pancreas, more than 2 cm in greatest dimension
T3   Tumour extends directly into any of the following: duodenum,
      bile duct, peripancreatic tissues
T4   Tumour extends directly into any of the following: stomach, spleen,
      colon, adjacent large vessels

Regional Lymph Nodes (N)
NX   Regional lymph nodes cannot be assessed
N0   No regional lymph node metastasis
N1   Regional lymph node metastasis
      N1a Metastasis in a single regional lymph node
      N1b Metastasis in multiple regional lymph nodes

Distant Metastasis (M)
MX   Distant metastasis cannot be assessed
M0   No distant metastasis
M1   Distant metastasis

Stage Grouping*

Stage	T	N	M
Stage 0	Tis	N0	M0
Stage I	T1	N0	M0
	T2	N0	M0
Stage II	T3	N0	M0
Stage III	T1	N1	M0
	T2	N1	M0
	T3	N1	M0
Stage IV A	T4	Any N	M0
Stage IV A	Any T	Any N	M1

* Information should be provided about the absence (R0 – no residual tumor detected) or the presence (R1 – microscopic residual tumour; R2 – macroscopic residual tumour) of residual tumour after resection.
[#] UICC TNM Classification of Malignant Tumors, 5th edition 1997, Wiley-Liss, New York.

incidence between the ages of 60 and 80, and is very rare in patients younger than 40. Most tumours occur in the head of the pancreas and have already invaded the peripancreatic tissue at the time of diagnosis.

Histological grading of ductal adenocarcinoma into well-, moderately and poorly differentiated groups has been found to be of prognostic significance. The grading criteria which consider the cytological and architectural features of the carcinoma are described in the "Explanatory Notes" (see Sect. 1.3.2) and are summarised in Table 2.

The most widely recognised staging system of ductal adenocarcinoma is that proposed by the International Union Against Cancer (UICC) in 1987 (see Table 3). It is based on the size and extent of the primary tumour (T), the status of the regional lymph nodes (N), and of metastatic disease (M).

Histological Classification of Tumours of the Exocrine Pancreas

1   **Epithelial Tumours**

1.1	*Benign*	
1.1.1	Serous cystadenoma	8441/0[a]
1.1.2	Mucinous cystadenoma	8470/0
1.1.3	Intraductal papillary-mucinous adenoma	8503/0
1.1.4	Mature teratoma	9080/0
1.2	*Borderline (Uncertain Malignant Potential)*	
1.2.1	Mucinous cystic tumour with moderate dysplasia	8470/1
1.2.2	Intraductal papillary-mucinous tumour with moderate dysplasia	8503/1
1.2.3	Solid-pseudopapillary tumour	8452/1
1.3	*Malignant*	
1.3.1	Severe ductal dysplasia/carcinoma in situ	8500/2
1.3.2	Ductal adenocarcinoma	8500/3
1.3.2.1	Mucinous noncystic carcinoma	8480/3
1.3.2.2	Signet-ring cell carcinoma	8490/3
1.3.2.3	Adenosquamous carcinoma	8560/3
1.3.2.4	Undifferentiated (anaplastic) carcinoma	8021/3
1.3.2.5	Mixed ductal-endocrine carcinoma	8154/3
1.3.3	Osteoclast-like giant cell tumour	8030/3
1.3.4	Serous cystadenocarcinoma	8441/3
1.3.5	Mucinous cystadenocarcinoma	8470/3
1.3.5.1	Noninvasive	8470/2
1.3.5.2	Invasive	8470/3

---

[a] Morphology code of the International Classification of Diseases for Oncology (ICD-O) and the Systematized Nomenclature of Medicine (SNOMED).

Definitions and Explanatory Notes

1 Epithelial Tumours

1.1 Benign

1.1.1 Serous cystadenoma (Figs. 1–3)

A benign cystic tumour composed of cuboidal epithelium producing serous fluid.

This tumour consists of multiple cysts lined by cuboidal or flattened epithelial cells which occasionally form small papillary infoldings. The cytoplasm of the cuboidal cells is pale to clear and only rarely eosinophilic. PAS staining without diastase digestion may be positive due to the presence of intracytoplasmic glycogen. There is no epithelial dysplasia. The cysts are separated by hyalinized septa which may contain entrapped islets. Grossly, two types of serous cystadenomas can be distinguished: *serous microcystic adenoma*, which is more common, and *serous oligocystic adenoma*.

The *serous microcystic adenoma* is a well-demarcated tumour composed of numerous small cysts arranged around a central stellate scar. The central stellate scar is a dense fibrous core within the tumour, which may be calcified and from which fibrous trabeculae radiate to the periphery. The tumour occurs predominantly in women.

The *serous oligocystic adenoma* is an often ill-demarcated tumour composed of a few cysts showing diameters between 1 and 2 cm. Serous cystic tumours showing larger cysts have been referred to as serous macrocystic adenoma. The cysts may extend deeply into the surrounding pancreatic tissue. The tumour occurs equally in both sexes.

1.1.2 Mucinous cystadenoma (Figs. 4–5)

A benign cystic tumour composed of columnar mucin-producing epithelium supported by "ovarian-type" stroma.

This usually unilocular tumour is lined by a single layer of tall columnar epithelial cells. They stain for mucin, have a polarized nucleus and lack significant dysplastic changes or mitoses. Papillary infoldings and scattered endocrine cells may be found. The inner layer of the wall is composed of cellular connective tissue that resembles ovarian stroma; the outer wall consists of hyalinized connective tissue. This rare cystic tumour occurs preferentially in the body and tail of the pancreas and, in most cases, has no communication with the duct system. It is almost exclusively found in women. Transformation into a borderline tumour or a mucinous cystadenocarcinoma can occur (see Sect. 1.2.1: mucinous cystic tumour with moderate dysplasia; and Sect. 1.3.5: mucinous cystadenocarcinoma).

1.1.3 Intraductal papillary-mucinous adenoma (Fig. 6)

A benign intraductal papillary growth of neoplastic columnar cells producing mucin.

The normal duct epithelium is replaced by papillary proliferations of mucin-producing columnar epithelium which may contain some goblet-like cells and endocrine cells. The neoplastic epithelium forms papillae of varying sizes which are branched and have a fibrovascular stalk. There is no significant cellular atypia and mitoses are almost absent. In the mucin-hypersecreting tumours the papillary projections are usually small and macroscopically not visible. This tumour usually originates from the main pancreatic duct, but may also primarily develop in one of the secondary ducts. It may present as a grossly circumscribed intraductal mass (papilloma) or as multiple small intraductal proliferations involving a large area of the duct system. In the latter case the intraductal epithelial proliferations are hardly visible grossly, but produce such a large amount of mucin that the involved ducts are cystically dilated. The nontumorous pancreatic tissue upstream of the involved duct segment is usually fibrotic due to obstructive pancreatitis. Transformation into a borderline tumour or an intraductal papillary-mucinous carcinoma may occur (see Sect. 1.2.2: intraductal papillary-mucinous tumour with moderate dysplasia; and Sect. 1.3.6: intraductal papillary-mucinous carcinoma).

This lesion has also been referred to by numerous other terms such as mucin-producing tumour, mucin-hypersecreting tumour, mucinous ductal ectasia, duct ectatic type of pancreatic ductal carcinoma, diffuse villous carcinoma and villous adenoma. Since these terms either do not properly reflect the complex nature of the lesion or may lead to confusion with other pancreatic tumours, we selected the name "intraductal papillary-mucinous tumour".

1.1.4 Mature teratoma

A benign extragonadal germ cell tumour with mature tissue derived from all three germinal layers.

This tumour has usually been referred to as dermoid cyst. It appears as a unilocular or multilocular cystic neoplasm. It is classified among the epithelial tumors for convenience, as it always contains an epithelial element.

1.2 Borderline (Uncertain Malignant Potential)

1.2.1 Mucinous cystic tumour with moderate dysplasia
(Fig. 7)

A cystic tumour composed of columnar mucin-producing epithelium that shows moderately dysplastic changes and is supported by "ovarian-type stroma". The tumour may transform into a mucinous cystadenocarcinoma, but usually behaves as a benign neoplasm if properly treated.

The cystic tumour may be unilocular or multilocular. The lining columnar cells are commonly admixed with goblet-like cells and single endocrine cells. They form papillary infoldings and display foci of moderate dysplasia characterized by cellular pseudostratification with crowding of nuclei. Most nuclei are still basally located but tend to be irregular in size. Mitoses occur. The subepithelial stroma is composed of cellular connective tissue that resembles ovarian stroma and may contain crypt-like invaginations of the columnar epithelium or groups of daughter glands without significant atypia. Unequivocal stromal invasion by frankly atypical glands is absent. Like mucinous cystadenoma, the tumour occurs preferentially in the body and tail of the pancreas, lacks communication with the duct system in most cases and is almost exclusively found in women.

1.2.2 Intraductal papillary-mucinous tumour with moderate dysplasia (Fig. 8)

An intraductal papillary growth of neoplastic columnar cells producing mucin and showing foci of moderate dysplasia. The tumour may transform into an intraductal papillary-mucinous carcinoma.

Apart from more irregularly structured papillae and the presence of a moderately dysplastic epithelium, the features of borderline tumours are similar to those of the intraductal papillary-mucinous adenoma (see Sect. 1.1.3). The papillary epithelium showing moderate dysplasia is characterized by slightly irregularly sized and hyperchromatic polarized nuclei, with an occasional distinct nucleolus, nuclear crowding and stratification, and variable mucin content. Mitoses are relatively frequent. Severe dysplastic changes or carcinoma in situ, however, are absent.

1.2.3 Solid-pseudopapillary tumour (Figs. 9–13)

An epithelial tumour composed of monomorphous cells forming solid and pseudopapillary structures, frequently with haemorrhagic-cystic changes. The tumour usually has a benign behaviour, but occasionally may be malignant.

This tumour has also been referred to as solid and papillary epithelial neoplasm, solid and cystic tumour, and papillary and cystic tumour. The tumour tissue displays a solid and focally pseudopapillary pattern, with variable stromal sclerosis. In both patterns, the monomorphous tumour cells are arranged around delicate and often hyalinized fibrovascular stalks. The tumour cells have a round to oval nucleus and a slightly eosinophilic or clear cytoplasm, which may contain diastase-resistant PAS-positive globules. Mitoses are rare. Scattered groups of foam cells or degenerative changes such as tissue haemorrhage with pseudocystic transformation and cholesterol crystals surrounded by foreign body cells are commonly seen. The tumours are usually well demarcated from the adjoining pancreatic tissue and invasion into the surrounding parenchyma is rare. The capsular tissue may contain calcifications. Young women are predominantly affected.

1.3 Malignant

1.3.1 Severe ductal dysplasia/carcinoma in situ (Fig. 14)

A change of the ductal epithelium characterised by irregular epithelial budding and bridging, and severe nuclear abnormalities such as loss of polarity, pleomorphism, coarse chromatin, dense nucleoli and mitotic figures. This lesion can be considered as noninvasive ductal adenocarcinoma.

Severe ductal dysplasia/carcinoma in situ changes usually occur in medium-sized ducts. The epithelial lining of the involved duct is irregular, displaying pseudostratification, small papillae with bridging, and irregular projections lacking fibrovascular stalks. The nuclei show marked abnormalities. The lesion is often surrounded by one or two layers of fibrosclerotic tissue. It cannot be recognized by gross examination.

Severe ductal dysplasia/carcinoma in situ changes are commonly found in association with an invasive ductal adenocarcinoma. Usually they are observed immediately adjacent to the invasive carcinoma. Occasionally, however, carcinoma in situ changes may also be seen remote from the invasive tumour. Some investigators regard the latter finding as evidence for multicentric cancer development, while others consider them continuous intraductal extensions of the invasive tumour. Severe dysplasia/carcinoma in situ changes have only rarely been observed in an otherwise normal pancreas.

No attempt is made to distinguish between severe dysplasia and carcinoma in situ, since it is very difficult, if not impossible, to draw a clear distinction between these two changes.

Severely dysplastic acinar changes have not yet been described.

1.3.2 Ductal adenocarcinoma (Figs. 15–19)

A carcinoma composed of mucin-producing glands resembling normal pancreatic duct structures.

This tumour is the most common form of pancreatic carcinoma. It accounts for 80%–85% of all cases. The tumour glands show varying degrees of severe cytological atypia, are often well developed, produce various amounts of mucin, elicit a desmoplastic reaction and invade the stroma.

Ductal adenocarcinoma can be divided into well-, moderately and poorly differentiated types. The well-differentiated carcinomas show relatively large duct-like structures combined with medium-sized tubular and occasionally cribriform neoplastic glands, which are irregularly arranged within a desmoplastic stroma. Between the neoplastic glands there may be a few nonneoplastic ducts as well as remnants of acini and islets. The neoplastic duct-like glands may be so well differentiated that they are difficult to distinguish from nonneoplastic ducts. Commonly they contain single endocrine cells which stain for pancreatic hormones. The mucin-producing tumour cells tend to be columnar, display an eosinophilic and occasionally pale or clear cytoplasm, and contain round to oval nuclei which vary in size and have a distinct nucleolus. Extension into the adjoining pancreatic tissue occurs via the interlobular septa or preexisting ducts (see Sect. 1.3.1: severe dysplasia/carcinoma in situ changes).

The moderately differentiated carcinomas show predominantly medium-sized duct-like and tubular structures of various shapes which are embedded in desmoplastic stroma and completely replace the acinar tissue. Compared with the well-differentiated carcinoma there is a much greater degree of cellular atypia and more mitotic figures are seen.

The poorly differentiated carcinomas are composed of a mixture of densely packed, small irregular glands as well as solid tumour cell sheets and nests, which entirely replace the acinar tissue. Foci of squamoid differentiation or complete anaplasia (comprising less than 20% of the tumour tissue) may occur. Usually there is only little desmoplasia, but necrotic and haemorrhagic changes may be present. The tumour cells display a high degree of pleomorphism, reduced mucin production, and many mitotic figures.

A ductal adenocarcinoma showing various degrees of differentiation should be classified according to the least differentiated part (see also Table 2).

From 60% to 70% of ductal adenocarcinomas are localised in the head of the pancreas. They occur somewhat more frequently in men than in women, and are extremely rare before the age of 40.

1.3.2.1   Mucinous noncystic carcinoma (Fig. 20)

An adenocarcinoma composed of well-differentiated glands with abundant extracellular mucin production.

More than 50% of the tumour tissue consists of mucin. This gives the carcinoma a gelatinous or colloid cut surface, but does not result in cystic changes. Apart from some duct-like glands the tumour shows mucin lakes which are partly lined by well-differentiated columnar epithelium and contain floating clumps or strands of tumour cells. The relative frequency of this rare tumour is 1%–3%.

1.3.2.2 Signet-ring cell carcinoma (Figs. 21, 22)

An adenocarcinoma composed almost exclusively of mucin-filled signet-ring cells.

This tumour exhibits a markedly infiltrative spread and may involve almost the entire pancreas, resulting in diffuse enlargement of the gland. The relative frequency is less than 1%.

1.3.2.3 Adenosquamous carcinoma (Fig. 23)

A carcinoma composed of a mixture of neoplastic glandular and squamoid components.

The squamous component of this carcinoma should account for at least 30% of the tumour tissue and may show variable differentiation. In areas with an intimate intermingling of glandular and squamoid components the tumour displays a mucoepidermoid pattern. A pure squamous carcinoma might be possible, but extensive sampling usually reveals some neoplastic glands in the squamoid component. In metastases, the adenocarcinoma component may be the only pattern present. The relative frequency of this rare tumour is 3%–4%.

1.3.2.4 Undifferentiated (anaplastic) carcinoma (Figs. 24–27)

A carcinoma composed of pleomorphic large cells, giant cells and/or spindle cells.

This tumour has been referred to as giant cell carcinoma, pleomorphic large cell carcinoma and sarcomatoid carcinoma. It resembles a sarcoma, but immunohistologically the neoplastic cells stain for cytokeratin and commonly also for vimentin. Foci of glandular differentiation may be found in many of these tumours after extensive sampling. Undifferentiated carcinomas with a neoplastic mesenchymal component (carcinosarcoma) have not yet been observed. The tumour may be large and partly necrotic. Its frequency ranges from 2%–7%.

1.3.2.5 Mixed ductal-endocrine carcinoma (Fig. 28)

A carcinoma in which ductal and endocrine cells are intimately admixed.

The endocrine cell component should comprise at least 30% of the tumour tissue. The endocrine cells are characterised by their expression of general neuroendocrine markers, the ductal cells by mucin production and carcinoembryonic antigen. The behaviour is dictated by the ductal component. These tumours are extremely rare (<1%).

1.3.3 Osteoclast-like giant cell tumour (Figs. 29–30)

A tumour composed of undifferentiated epithelial and/or mesenchymal cells admixed with nonneoplastic osteoclast-like giant cells.

These tumours show two cell populations, neoplastic spindle-shaped to pleomorphic cells and nonneoplastic osteoclast-like giant cells usually containing more than 20 uniformly small nuclei. In addition, there may be foci of neoplastic ductal glands. Osteoid formation may also occur. The neoplastic cells stain immunohistochemically for cytokeratin and/or vimentin, the osteolast-like cells for leukocyte-common antigen. The tumour may arise in association with a mucinous cystadenocarcinoma. The frequency is <1%.

1.3.4 Serous cystadenocarcinoma (Fig. 31)

A low-grade cystic carcinoma composed of cuboidal cells producing serous fluid.

This extremely rare tumour resembles serous cystadenoma but shows invasive and metastatic growth.

1.3.5 Mucinous cystadenocarcinoma (Figs. 32, 33)

A cystic carcinoma composed of (at least focally) severely dysplastic columnar epithelium producing mucin and supported by ovarian-type stroma.

This is a unilocular or multilocular cystic tumour which shows severe dysplasia/carcinoma in situ changes, commonly in addition to foci of less severe dysplasia. The severely dysplastic areas are characterised by papillae with irregular branching and budding, and nuclear stratification with severe nuclear abnormalities as well as frequent mitosis. Apart from typical ovarian-type stroma the wall of the lesion displays haemorrhage, calcification and/or chronic inflammation, sometimes with foreign-body-type reaction. This is often seen in relation to mucin spillage from ruptured cysts. Rarely does the cyst wall contain pseudosarcomatous or frankly sarcomatous nodules. According to the absence or presence of stromal invasion of fibrous septa and the cyst wall by neoplastic glands, the *noninvasive* (8470/2) or *invasive type* (8470/3) of mucinous cystadenocarcinoma must be differentiated. If an invasive component is present, it resembles the usual ductal adenocarcinoma or one of its variants.

1.3.6 Intraductal papillary-mucinous carcinoma (Figs. 34–37)

An intraductal carcinoma composed of papillary proliferations of severely dysplastic mucin-producing epithelium.

This tumour shows irregular papillary infoldings which are lined, at least partly, by markedly atypical epithelium. Apart from nuclear abnormalities (i.e. nuclear pleomorphism, conspicuous nucleoli, mitotic figures) the atypical epithelium may form small irregular papillae which are not supported by fibrovascular tissue stalks and may display a cribriform pattern. Due to intraductal tumour growth and usually also to mucin hypersecretion the involved ducts are cystically dilated. The neoplastic papillary epithelium often extends into secondary ducts, but remains confined within the duct system. According to the absence or presence of neoplastic glandular structures invading the pancreatic tissue surrounding the involved ducts the tumours must be separated into *noninvasive* (8503/2) and *invasive type* (8503/3) (*papillary-mucinous carcinoma*). Parenchymal invasion may be difficult to distinguish from secondary duct involvement. The invasive component resembles either the usual ductal adenocarcinoma or, what seems to be more common, the mucinous noncystic carcinoma.

1.3.7 Acinar cell carcinoma (Figs. 38–41)

A carcinoma composed of neoplastic acinar cells and an occasional component of endocrine cells.

This tumour shows markedly cellular tissue which is lobulated by fibrous strands. Typically, the tumour cells form an acinar ("microglandular") pattern, but a mixed pattern in which trabecular and solid formations alternate with acinar areas is more common. In some tumours acinar formations are (almost) absent. The tumour cells have relatively uniform round nuclei and a granular cytoplasm which may be diastase-resistant PAS-positive. Mitotic figures are common. Immunohistochemically, the tumour cells stain for pancreatic enzymes such as trypsin or lipase. In addition, there may be some scattered neoplastic endocrine cells or small endocrine cell clusters which stain for neuroendocrine markers such as synaptophysin and chromo-granin A, and pancreatic hormones.

The tumour is more frequent in men than women and may also occur in children or adolescents. The frequency is about 1%. A few acinar cell carcinomas present with subcutaneous fat necrosis and polyarthralgia. There are no convincing reports of acinar cell adenomas.

1.3.7.1 Acinar cell cystadenocarcinoma (Fig. 42)

An extrermely rare acinar cell carcinoma with multilocular cyst formation.

1.3.7.2 Mixed acinar-endocrine carcinoma

An acinar cell carcinoma with an endocrine component which comprises at least one third of the entire tumour cell population.

1.3.8 Pancreatoblastoma (Figs. 43–45)

A malignant tumour composed of epithelial tissue with acinar differentiation, squamoid cell nests and occasional endocrine cells.

These tumours, which are usually encapsulated, show lobules and nests of relatively uniform cells separated by dense fibrous stroma. The cells grow in acinar, glandular or more solid (i.e. undifferentiated) patterns which blend with scattered squamoid cell nests. Immunohistochemically, the acinar cells stain for pancreatic enzymes. In some tumours, there are scattered endocrine- or alpha foetoprotein (AFP)-positive cells.

Pancreatoblastomas occur typically in children and are only rarely observed in adults. A few have been described in patients with the Beckwith-Wiedemann syndrome. The relative fre-quency is <1%.

1.3.9 Solid-pseudopapillary carcinoma (Fig. 46)

A low-grade carcinoma composed of monomorphous cells form-ing solid and pseudopapillary structures.

The neoplasm is identical to the solid-pseudopapillary tumour (see Sect. 1.2.3), but in addition shows clear criteria of malignancy such as vascular and nerve sheath invasion, and/or metastasis to lymph nodes and the liver.

1.3.10 Miscellaneous carcinomas

Among the miscellaneous carcinomas, which are all extremely rare, are clear cell carcinoma, ciliated cell carcinoma, oncocytic carcinoma, choriocarcinoma and nonmucinous, glycogen-poor cystadenocarcinoma.

2 Nonepithelial Tumours

All nonepithelial tumours of the pancreas described to date are much more common in extrapancreatic locations. Among the benign are granular cell tumour, fibrous histiocytoma, juvenile haemangioendothelioma and schwannoma. Among the malignant are leiomyosarcoma, malignant schwannoma, fibrosarcoma, malignant fibrous histiocytoma, liposarcoma, rhabdomyosarcoma and malignant haemangiopericytoma. The most frequent primary lymphoma encountered in the pancreas is extramedullary plasmacytoma. None of these tumours has a particular clinicopathological significance. As to the detailed definitions and explanatory notes, reference should be made to the WHO *Histological Typing of Soft Tissue Tumours.*

3 Secondary Tumours (Fig. 47)

Tumours that have extended directly or metastasized to the pancreas.

Secondary pancreatic tumours are uncommon and are usually discovered at autopsy. The tumours which most commonly spread haematogenously to the pancreas are lung carcinoma (especially small cell carcinoma), breast carcinoma, renal carcinoma, and melanoma. Secondary involvement of the pancreas by direct extension may be observed in ampullary carcinoma, signet-ring cell carcinoma of the stomach, colorectal carcinoma, peritoneal mesothelioma or abdominal lymphoma.

4 Tumour-like Lesions

4.1 Chronic pancreatitis (Figs. 48, 49)

A chronic inflammatory process characterized by duct changes, perilobular fibrosis and eventually panlobular scarring.

The ductal and ductular distortions and proliferations found in chronic pancreatitis may resemble well-differentiated ductal adenocarcinoma. However, in contrast to carcinoma, ducts and ductules in chronic pancreatitis retain their lobular arrangement and lack significant dysplastic changes such as nuclear pleomorphism, prominent nucleoli and mitotic figures. In addition, invasion of the nerve sheaths and the peripancreatic fatty tissue by atypical glands is absent in chronic pancreatitis. It must be emphasized that ductal carcinoma and chronic pancreatitis commonly occur together, because tumourous duct obstruction causes secondary chronic inflammation upstream of the stenosis. A diagnosis of primary chronic pancreatitis should be made with caution in a patient older than 60 years with increasing jaundice of short duration.

4.2 Miscellaneous inflammatory changes

Special forms of pancreatic inflammation include sarcoidosis and malakoplakia. The distinctive features of sarcoidosis are epithelioid granulomas. Malakoplakia is composed of macrophages, lymphocytes and plasma cells. The macrophages typically contain laminated calcified microspherules (Michaelis-Guttmann bodies).

4.3 Cysts

Tumour-like cystic lesions formed by nonneoplastic epithelial or mesenchymal cells.

4.3.1 Pseudocyst (Fig. 50)

A cyst filled with necrotic haemorrhagic debris rich in pancreatic enzymes and lined with granulation tissue.

Pseudocysts are usually found attached to the pancreas and are a consequence of an episode of acute pancreatitis.

4.3.2 Retention cyst

A cystic dilatation of a duct segment due to an obstruction by a stricture, stone (calculus) or mucin plug.

4.3.3 Parasitic cyst

A cystic mass caused by a parasite, namely Echinococcus.

4.3.4 Congenital cyst (Fig. 51)

Single or multiple thin-walled cysts lined by flattened non-neoplastic epithelial cells and containing serous fluid.

Congenital cysts are found as solitary lesions in the pancreas of infants and adults. If they are multiple, they are usually part of von Hippel-Lindau disease. Congenital cysts must be distinguished from serous cystadenoma.

4.3.5 Para-ampullary duodenal wall cyst (Fig. 52)

Single or multiple epithelial cysts in the submucosa and/or muscular layer of the duodenum in the vicinity of the ampulla of Vater. The cysts may be part of heterotopic pancreatic tissue.

Symptomatic para-ampullary duodenal wall cysts show intense inflammation which usually extends into the adjacent pancreatic and para-duodenal fatty tissue that is found between the duodenum and the distal common bile duct. The inflammatory process may lead to bile duct stenosis with symptoms mimicking carcinoma of the pancreas head. Whether the chronic and acute inflammation within and around the duodenal wall cysts are cause or consequence of the cystic transformation of ectopic pancreatic tissue is not known.

4.3.6 Enterogenous cyst

A cystic structure within or attached to the pancreas, representing a segmental duplication of the intestinal tract.

Enterogenous cysts are usually found in the duodenal wall. They are very rare and occur in children.

4.3.7 Lymphoepithelial cyst (Figs. 53, 54)

A unilocular cyst lined by mature squamoid epithelium which is supported by follicular lymphoid tissue.

Lymphoepithelial cysts may be large lesions which are found within or attached to the pancreas. Their structure is reminiscent of cervical branchial cysts. They occur predominantly in men.

4.3.8 Endometrial cyst

Ectopic endometrial tissue with cystic changes.

4.4 Duct changes

Alterations of the duct epithelium and the duct architecture which may be proliferative but do not show the criteria of severe dysplasia/carcinoma in situ (see Sect. 1.3.1).

There are four main changes of the pancreatic ducts: squamous metaplasia, mucinous cell hypertrophy, ductal papillary hyperplasia and adenomatoid ductal hyperplasia.

4.4.1 Squamous metaplasia (Fig. 55)

A focal lesion in which normal duct cells are replaced by squamous epithelium.

This lesion occurs in the normal as well as the chronically inflamed pancreas. It may be found in association with parasites entering the duct system or stenting of the main duct in chronic pancreatitis. Progression to squamous carcinoma has not yet been observed.

4.4.2 Mucinous cell hypertrophy (Fig. 56)

A focal lesion in which the normal duct epithelium is replaced by tall columnar mucin-filled cells lacking significant dysplastic changes.

This is a frequent lesion which has also been referred to as mucinous cell hyperplasia, mucoid transformation, mucinous cell metaplasia, goblet cell metaplasia, simple hyperplasia, non-papillary epithelial hypertrophy or ductal mucinous hyperplasia. It is found in the normal, the chronically inflamed and the nonneoplastic part of a pancreas that bears a tumour. Its frequency increases with age. The apical cytoplasm of the cells stains intensely with diastase-resistant PAS. The polarized nuclei appear to be normal in size or slightly enlarged. There are no mitoses. Mucinous cell hypertrophy in medium-sized ducts may be associated with *pyloric gland metaplasia* in small glands surrounding the larger duct.

4.4.3 Ductal papillary hyperplasia (Figs. 57, 58)

A focal lesion in which the normal duct epithelium is replaced by papillary folds lined by columnar cells displaying mucinous hypertrophy.

This is a frequent lesion which is found in the normal and the chronically inflamed pancreas as well as in association with a tumour. Its frequency increases with age. Due to papillary infolding of the epithelium the duct lumen may be obstructed, which causes acinar atrophy and lobular fibrosis upstream of the stenosis. Typically the papillary folds show a fibrovascular stalk. The nuclei are usually of larger size and their chromatin structure is more pronounced than those of the normal epithelium – criteria which can be interpreted as mild to moderate dysplasia. Mitotic figures, however, are not found. Ductal papillary hyperplasia is more frequent in the pancreas bearing an invasive ductal adenocarcinoma than in the normal pancreas. Although it is conceivable that ductal papillary hyperplasia may progress to carcinoma in situ, this transformation has not yet been convincingly demonstrated.

4.4.4 Adenomatoid ductal hyperplasia (Fig. 59)

This is a focal lesion consisting of an aggregation of small- to medium-sized ducts which usually show mucinous cell hypertrophy and pyloric gland metaplasia, and occasionally also ductal papillary hyperplasia.

This is a relatively rare lesion which is found in the normal and chronically inflamed pancreas as well as in association with a tumour. The lesion has an adenoma-like appearance, but often shows no sharp boundary and occasionally incorporates islets and some acini. There are no mitotic figures.

4.5 Acinar changes (Fig. 60)

Acinar cells can undergo tubular transformation, as in pancreatitis, or a focal alteration called acinar cell transforma-

tion, which has also been referred to as eosinophilic degenera-
tion of acinar cells, acinar cell dysplasia and hyperplastic acinar
cell nodule. In acinar cell transformation, the acinar cells acquire
a focal eosinophilic cytoplasm or a loss of basophilia. The size of
the cells and their nuclei is similar to that of the surrounding
acinar cells, but the nuclei may show a more dense chromatin or
be enlarged.

4.6 Heterotopic pancreas

*This is a focal lesion outside the pancreas consisting of heterotopic
(ectopic, aberrant) pancreatic tissue.*

Heterotopic pancreatic tissue is most commonly found in the
antrum of the stomach, the duodenum including the region of the
ampulla of Vater, the biliary tract and the jejunum. It is located
in the submucosa and/or the muscular layer. Typically the
heterotopic tissue includes all three components of the pancreas,
i.e. acini, ducts and islets. Occasionally, however, it is mainly
composed of ducts, with or without islets. The development of a
carcinoma in heterotopic pancreatic tissue seems to occur.

4.7 Heterotopic spleen

This lesion consists of ectopic splenic tissue within the pancreas.

4.8 Hamartoma

A hamartomatous change of the pancreas is a focal lesion consisting of disorderly arranged mature pancreatic tissue. It is composed of a mixture of ducts, acini and islets embedded in
abundant fibrotic stroma. A lobular architecture of the tissue is
missing. The hamartoma forms a grossly visible neoplastic ab-
normality. This lesion is extremely rare.

4.9 Inflammatory pseudotumour

An inflammatory pseudotumour is a nonneoplastic mass characterised by an admixture of inflammatory cells such as plasma

cells, lymphocytes, granulocytic cells and fibroblasts. Inflammatory pseudotumour is extremely rare.

4.10 Lipomatous pseudohypertrophy

A diffuse increase of the interstitial fatty tissue within the pancreas, which may lead to a marked enlargement of the gland.

4.11 Focal lymphoid hyperplasia

This rare focal lesion is a nonneoplastic aggregation of lymphoid tissue which resembles malignant lymphoma.

This focal change has also been referred to as pseudolymphoma. It is composed of a massive infiltration of lymphoid cells forming lymphoid follicles. The lymphocytes have been reported to be mature polyclonal B lymphocytes. The lesion may present as a mass.

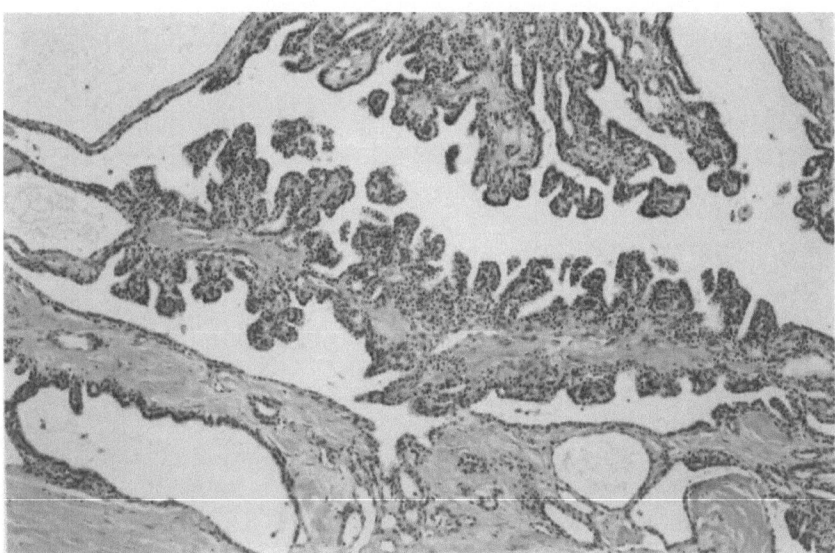

Fig. 1. *Serous cystadenoma, microcystic type.* The tumour tissue is composed of small cystic spaces lined by flat epithelial cells. The tumour is well demarcated from the adjacent pancreatic tissue

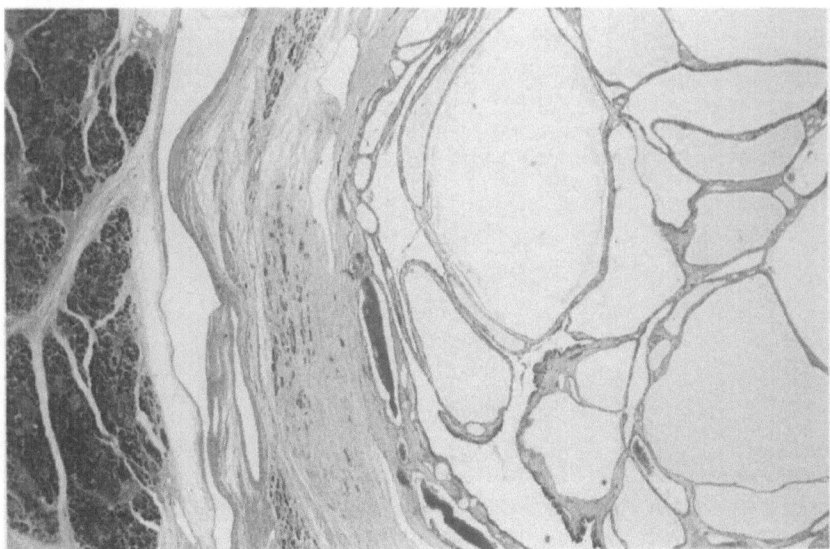

Fig. 2. *Serous cystadenoma, microcystic type.* The cuboidal cells lining the cysts may form papillary projections

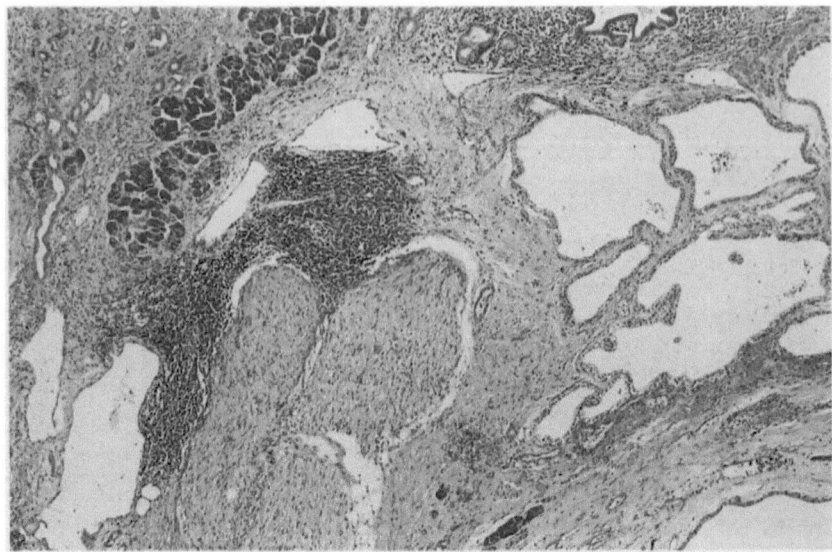

Fig. 3. *Serous cystadenoma, oligocystic type.* The cysts from the margin of the tumor extend into the adjacent pancreatic tissue

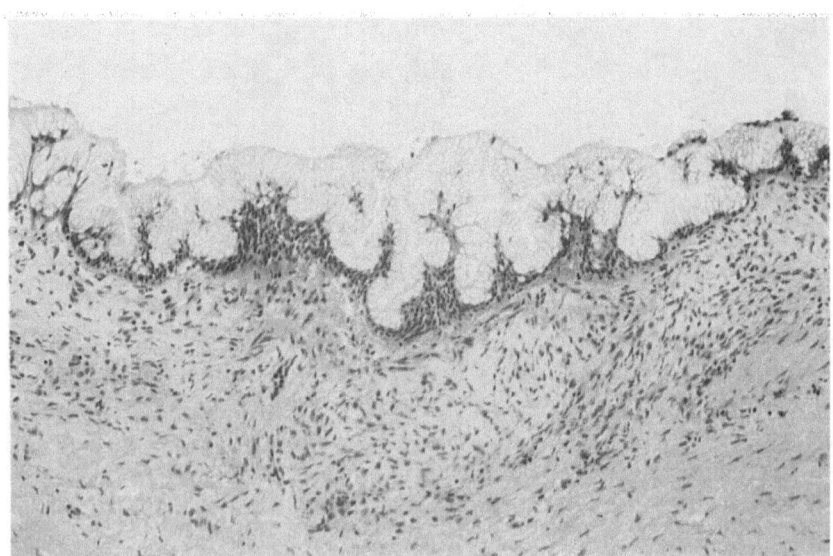

Fig. 4. *Mucinous cystadenoma.* The cyst is lined by a single layer of tall columnar cells which rest on a cellular mesenchymal stroma

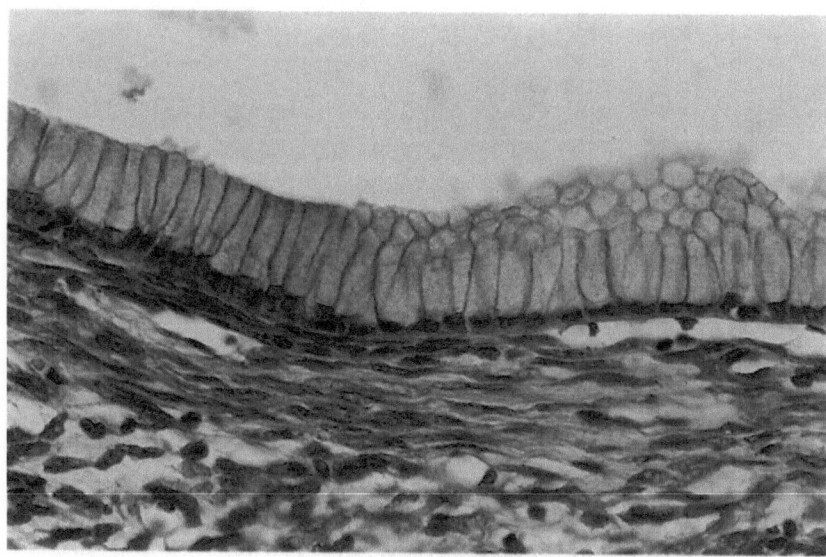

Fig. 5. *Mucinous cystadenoma.* The lining columnar cells show a uniformly sized nucleus which is located at the base of the cell. There are no significant dysplastic changes of the epithelium

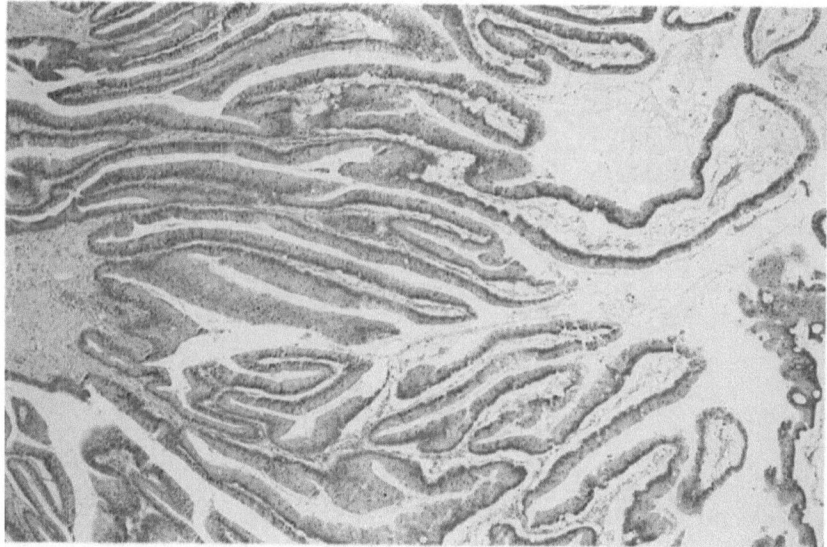

Fig. 6. *Intraductal papillary-mucinous adenoma.* The dilated pancreatic duct is partly filled with papillary epithelial proliferations which show a fibrovascular stalk and consist of tall columnar epithelial cells without any signs of significant atypia

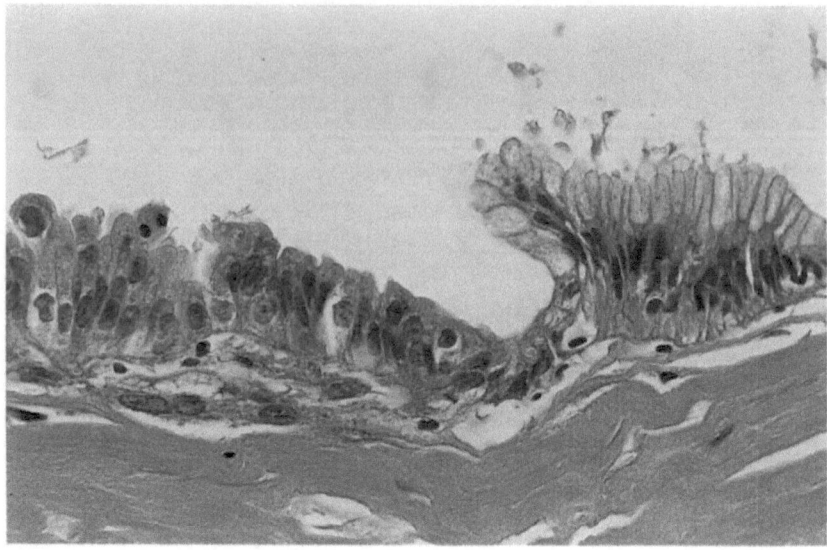

Fig. 7. *Mucinous cystic tumour with moderate dysplasia (borderline tumour).* The cyst-lining columnar epithelium shows moderate dysplasia characterized by cellular pseudostratification with crowding and enlarging of nuclei. Most nuclei, however, are still basally located

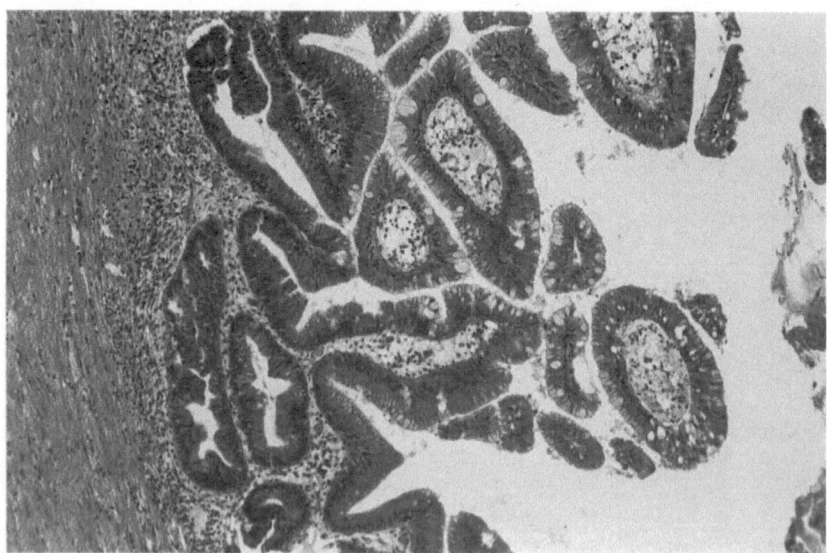

Fig. 8. *Intraductal papillary-mucinous tumour with moderate dysplasia (border-line tumour).* The papillary projections consist of columnar cells which are slightly irregularly sized and show hyperchromatic polarised nuclei

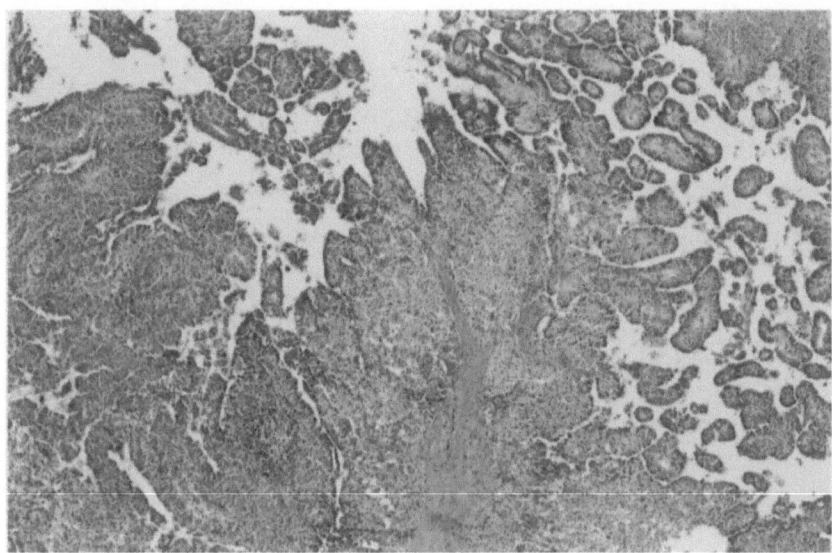

Fig. 9. *Solid-pseudopapillary tumour.* The tumour tissue shows a solid and partly pseudopapillary pattern

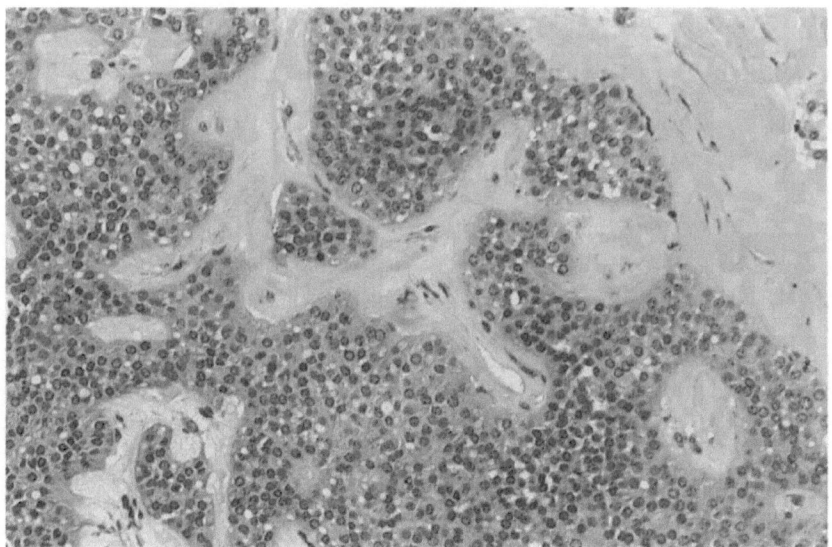

Fig. 10. *Solid-pseudopapillary tumour.* The tumour cells are monomorphous and arranged around delicate and often hyalinized fibrovascular stalks. The cytoplasm of the cells is slightly eosinophilic or clear

34

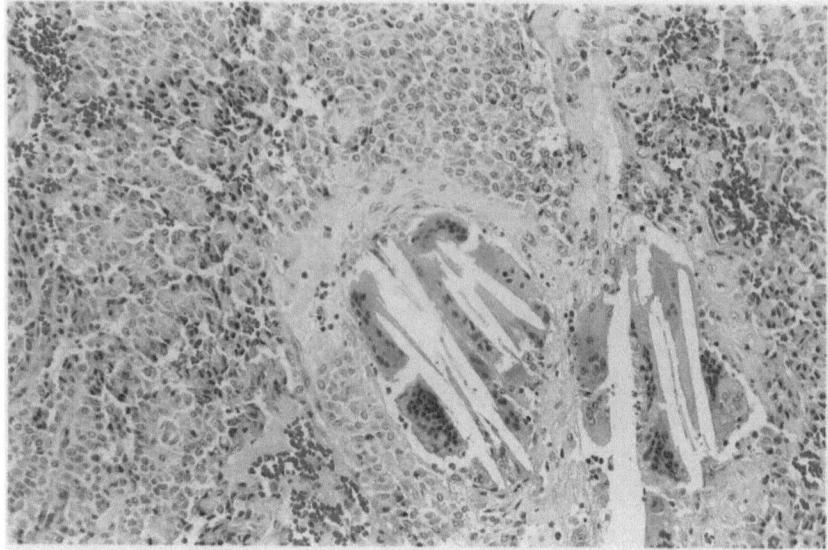

Fig. 11. *Solid-pseudopapillary tumour.* The solid tumour tissue includes cholesterol crystals surrounded by foreign body cells and hyalinized connective tissue

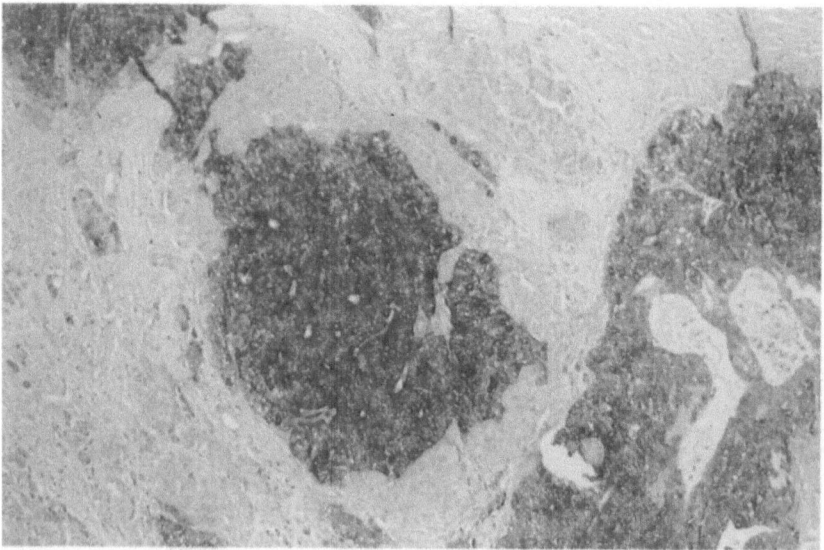

Fig. 12. *Solid-pseudopapillary tumour.* The tumour tissue shows intense immunostaining for neuron-specific enolase

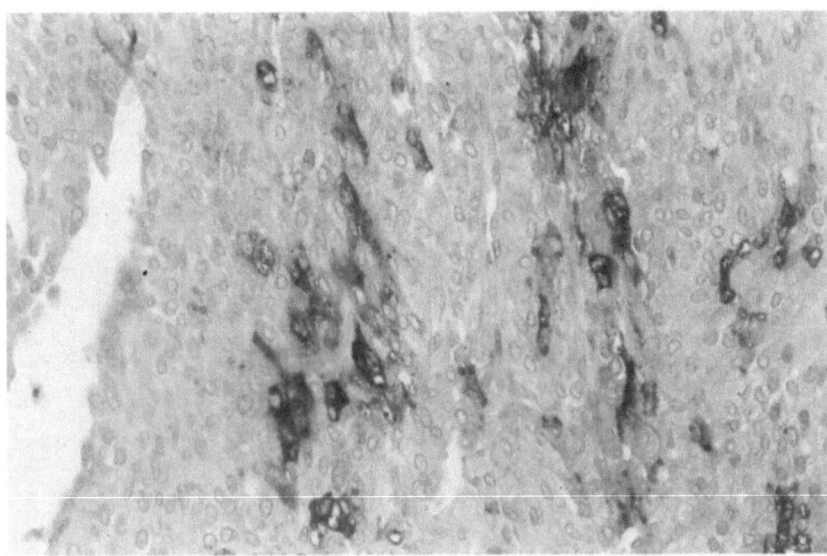

Fig. 13. *Solid-pseudopapillary tumour.* The tumour tissue shows intense focal immunostaining for alpha-1-anti-trypsin

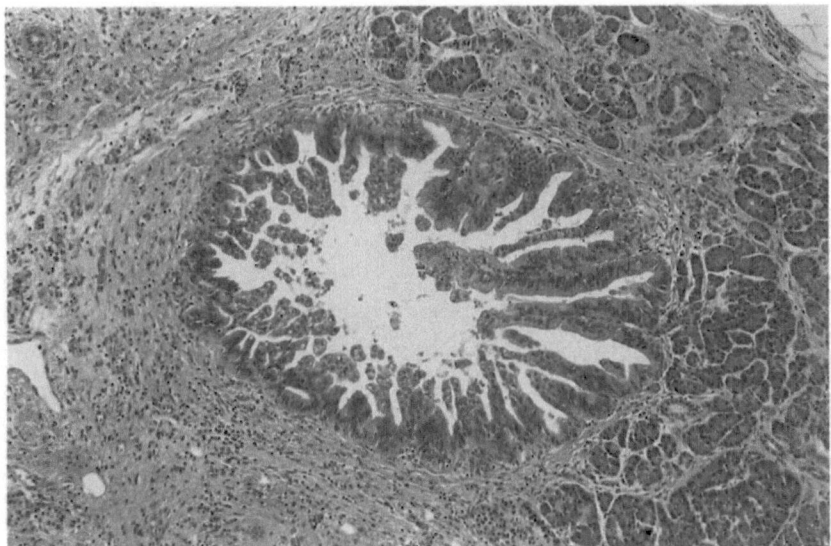

Fig. 14. *Severe ductal dysplasia/carcinoma in situ.* The epithelial lining of a medium-sized duct in the vicinity of an invasive ductal adenocarcinoma shows irregular cribriform projections lacking a fibrovascular stalk. In addition, there is distinct cellular atypia

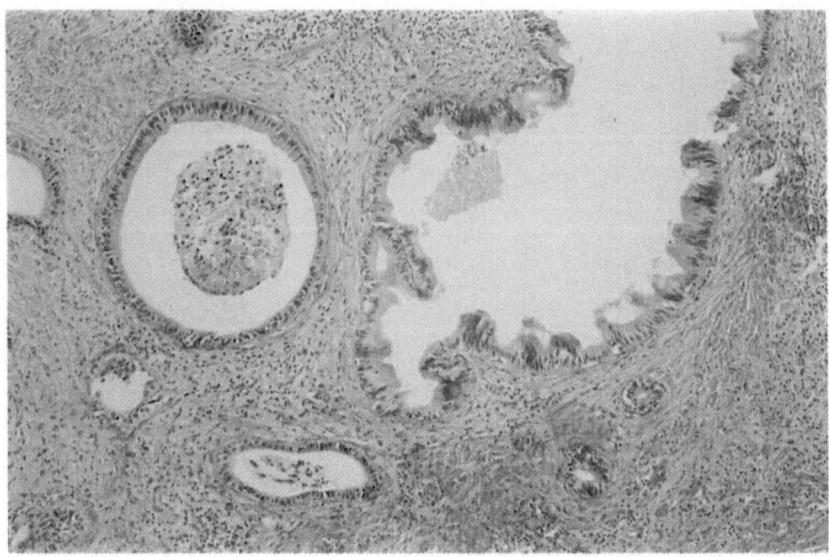

Fig. 15. *Ductal adenocarcinoma, well differentiated.* A low-power view of this ductal adenocarcinoma shows atypical duct-like structures and some smaller atypical tubular glands embedded in dense connective tissue

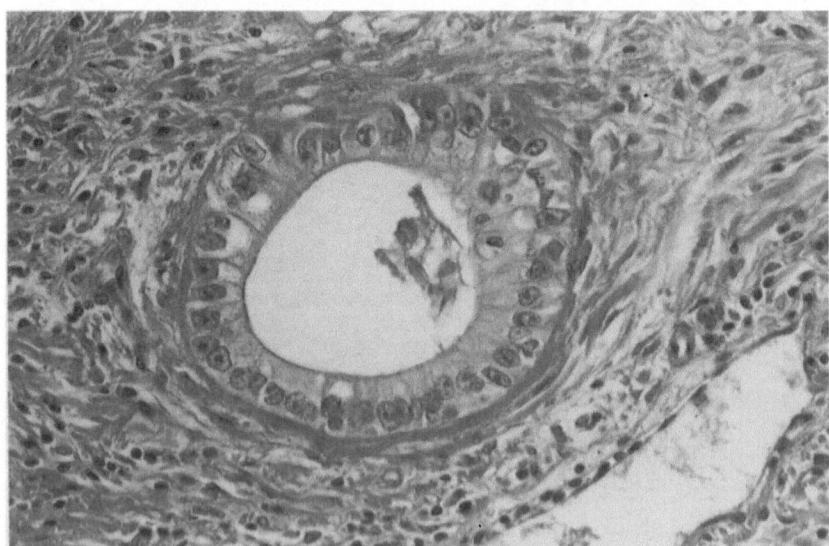

Fig. 16. *Ductal adenocarcinoma, well differentiated.* The neoplastic glands consist of mucin-producing columnar cells with little cellular atypia

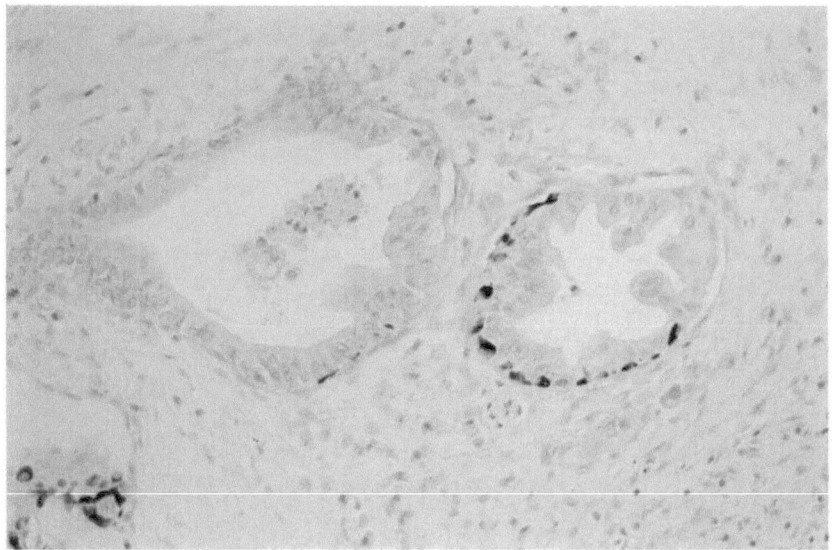

Fig. 17. *Ductal adenocarcinoma, well differentiated.* Immunostaining for glucagon reveals numerous endocrine cells attached to a neoplastic gland

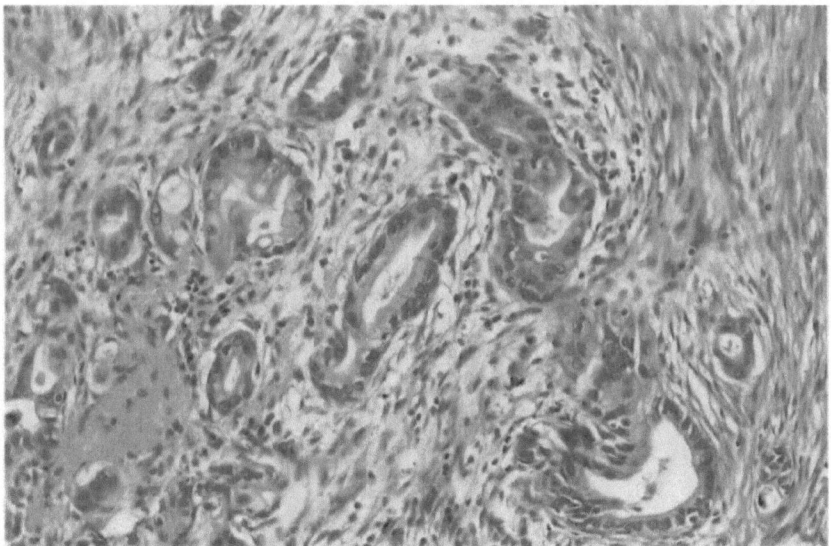

Fig. 18. *Ductal adenocarcinoma, moderately differentiated.* The neoplastic glands are irregularly shaped. The tumour cells show distinct cellular atypia

38

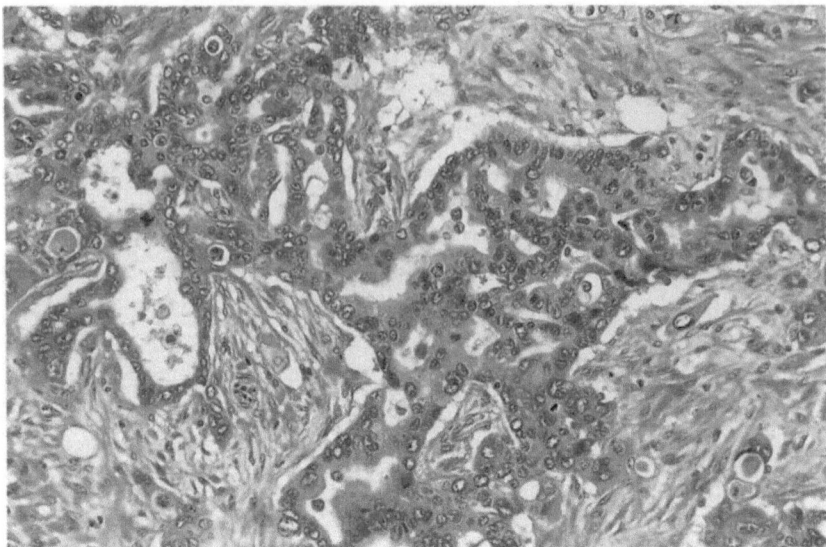

Fig. 19. *Ductal adenocarcinoma, poorly differentiated.* The tumour tissue is composed of completely irregularly shaped glands formed by severely atypical cells

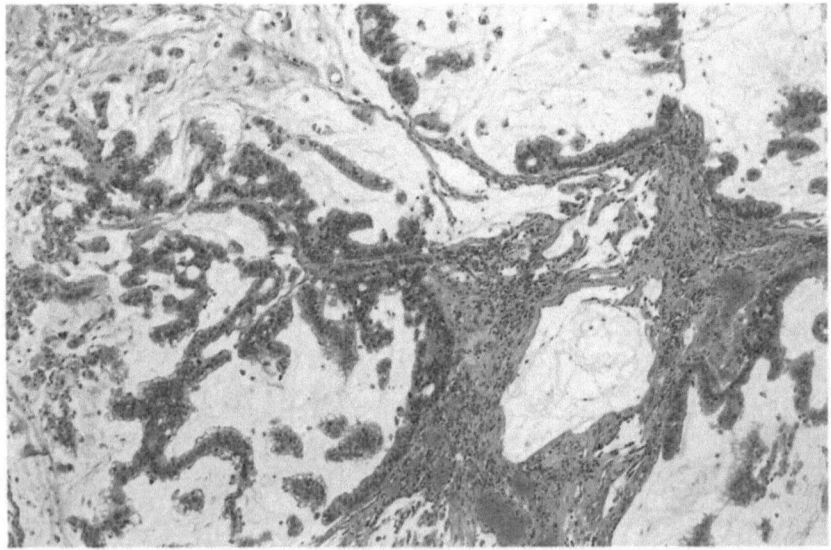

Fig. 20. *Mucinous noncystic carcinoma.* The tumour tissue shows a mucin lake which is partly lined by well-differentiated neoplastic columnar cells. In addition, there are single tumour cells floating free within the mucin

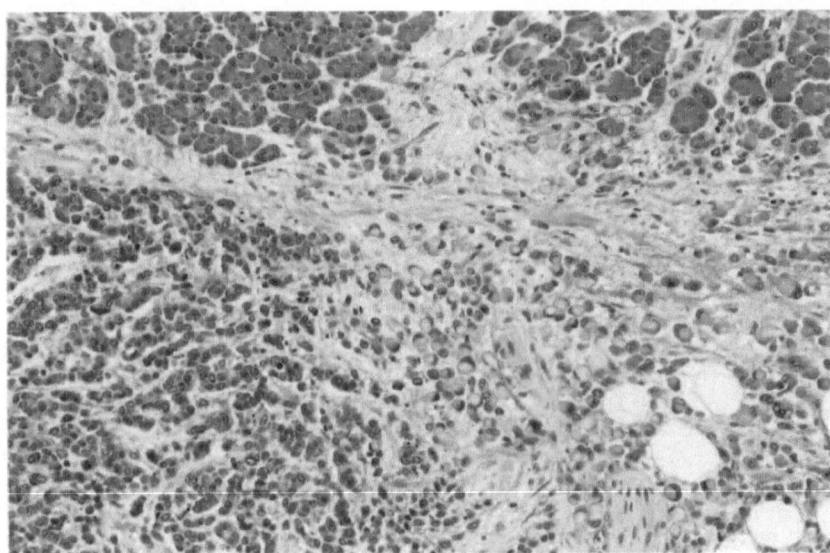

Fig. 21. *Signet-ring cell carcinoma.* The pancreatic tissue shows diffuse invasion by signet-ring carcinoma cells

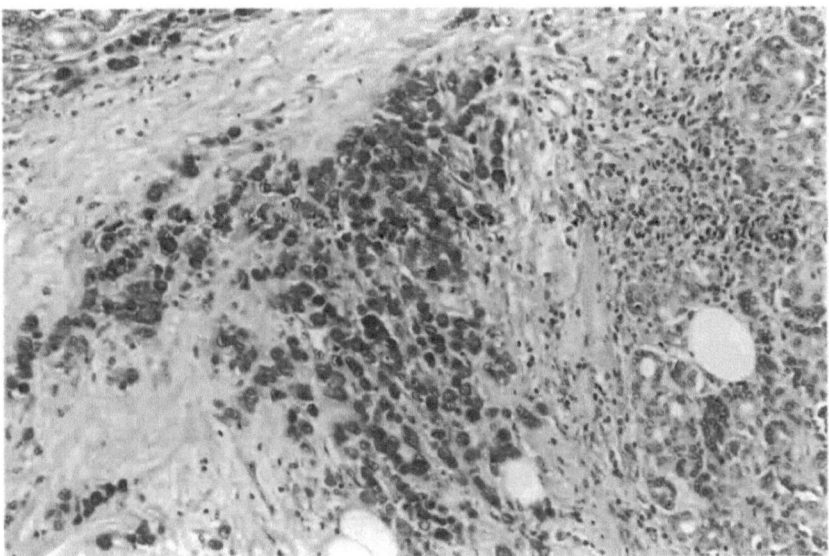

Fig. 22. *Signet-ring cell carcinoma.* PAS staining reveals the mucin content of the tumour cells

40

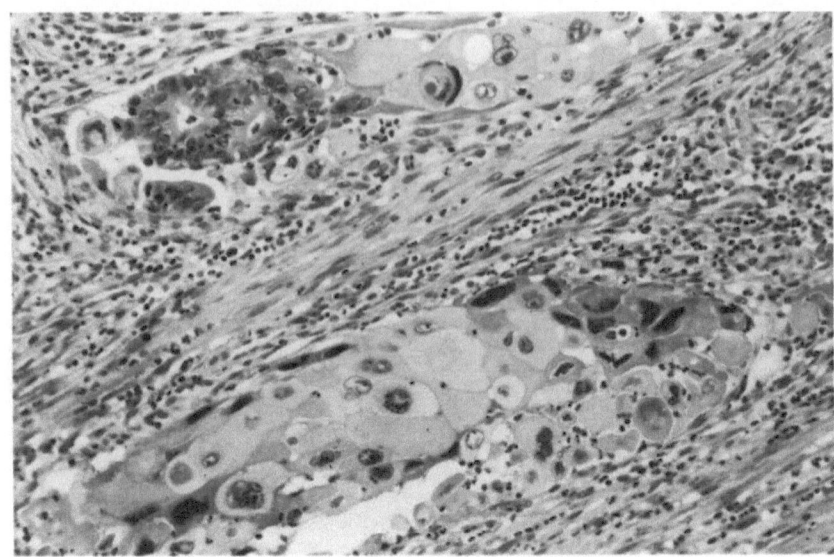

Fig. 23. *Adenosquamous carcinoma*. The tumour tissue shows an intimate intermingling of glandular and squamoid components

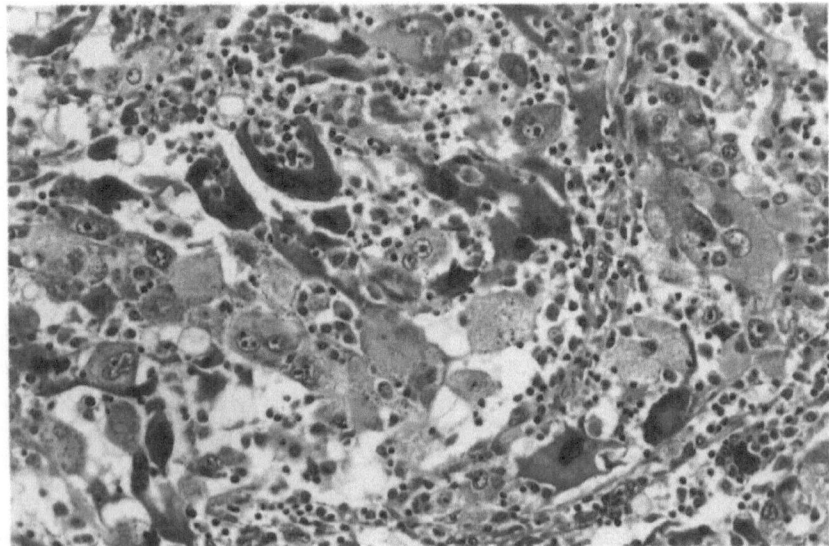

Fig. 24. *Undifferentiated (anaplastic) carcinoma*. The tumour tissue is composed of pleomorphic large cells and some giant cells

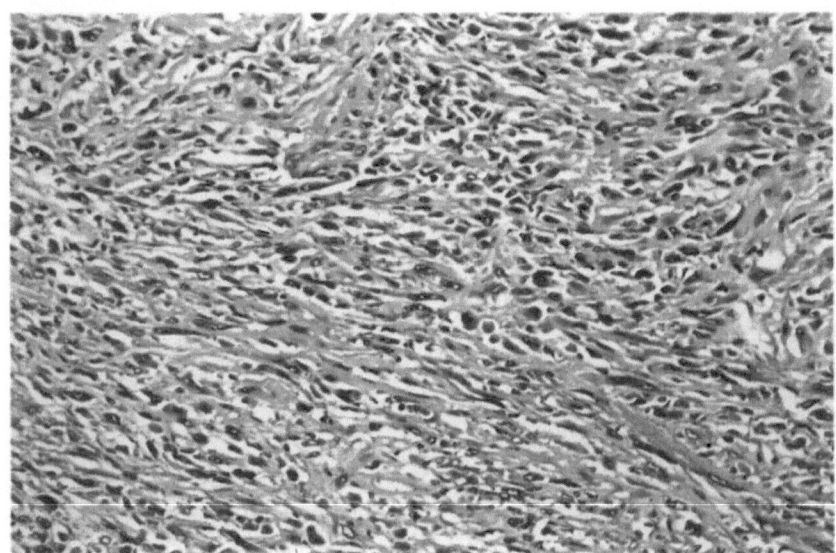

Fig. 25. *Undifferentiated (anaplastic) carcinoma.* The tumour tissue is composed of spindle cells

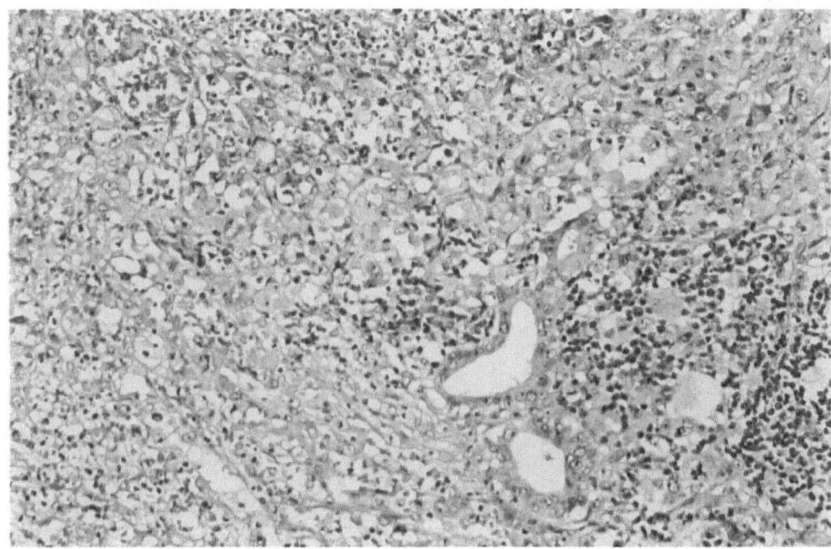

Fig. 26. *Undifferentiated (anaplastic) carcinoma.* The tumour tissue shows a focus of glandular differentiation

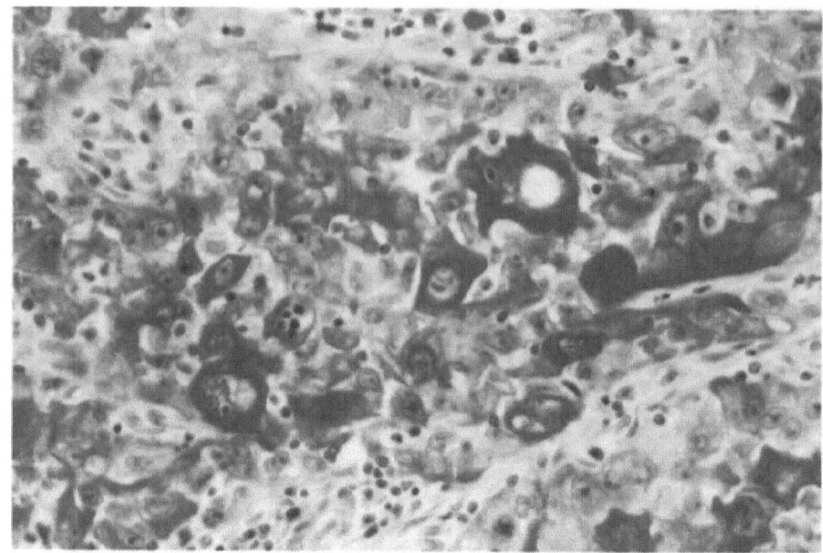

Fig. 27. *Undifferentiated (anaplastic) carcinoma.* Immunostaining for cyto-keratin (CK19) reveals strong positivity of pleomorphic tumour cells

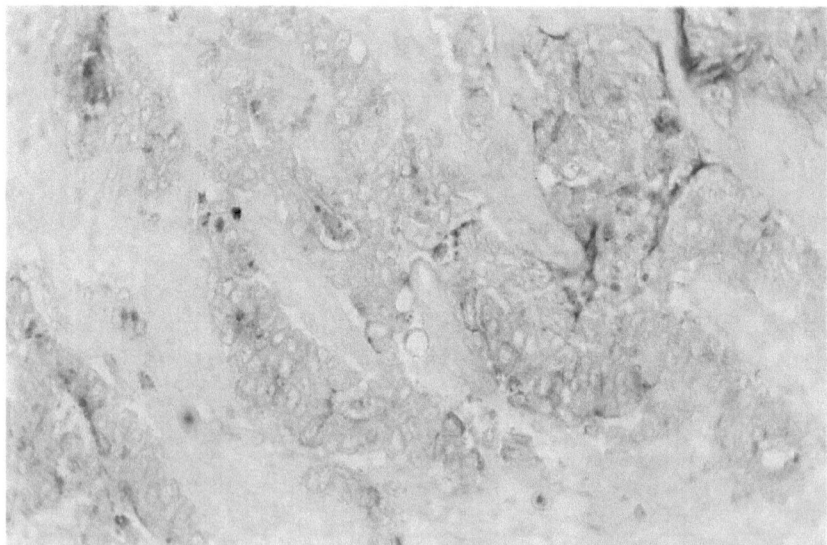

Fig. 28. *Mixed ductal-endocrine carcinoma.* Immunolabelling for syn-aptophysin combined with PAS staining reveals endocrine cells as well as mucin-producing cells forming small glands

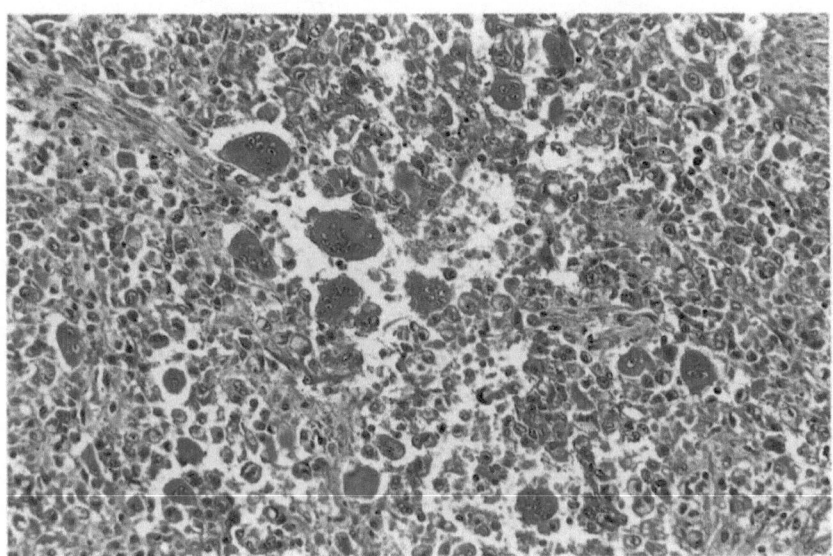

Fig. 29. *Osteoclast-like giant cell tumour.* The tumour tissue is composed of pleomorphic tumour cells which are intermingled with nonneoplastic osteoclast-like giant cells

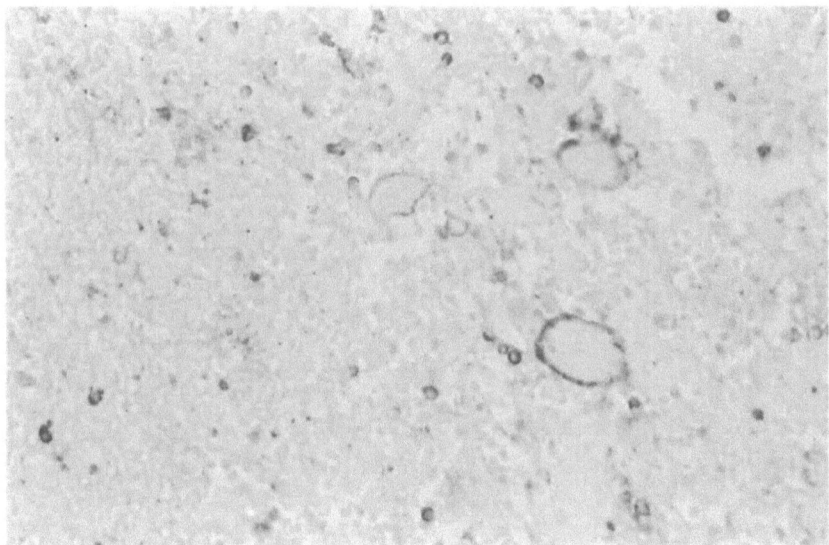

Fig. 30. *Osteoclast-like giant cell tumour.* Immunostaining for leukocyte common antigen shows membraneous labelling of osteoclast-like cells and some scattered lymphocytes. The neoplastic cells remain negative

44

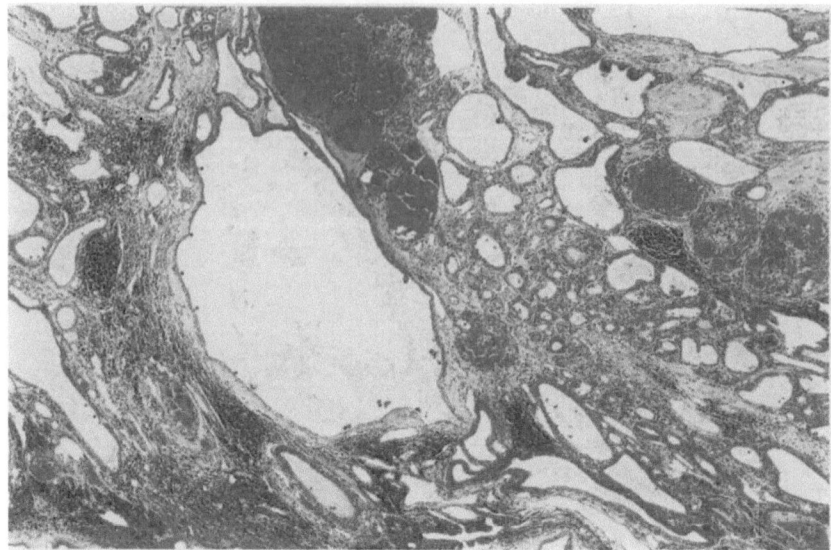

Fig. 31. *Serous cystadenocarcinoma.* Metastatic tumour tissue in a lymph node

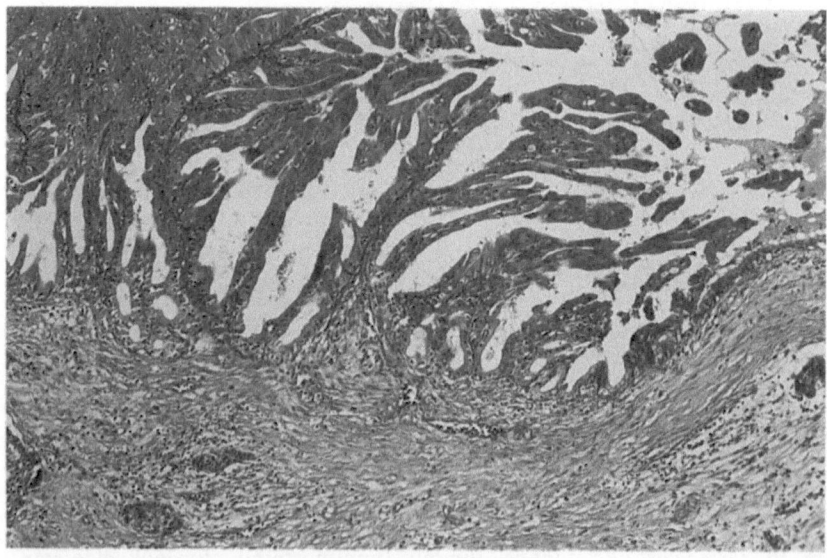

Fig. 32. *Mucinous cystadenocarcinoma.* The cyst is lined by severely atypical columnar cells forming irregular papillary projections

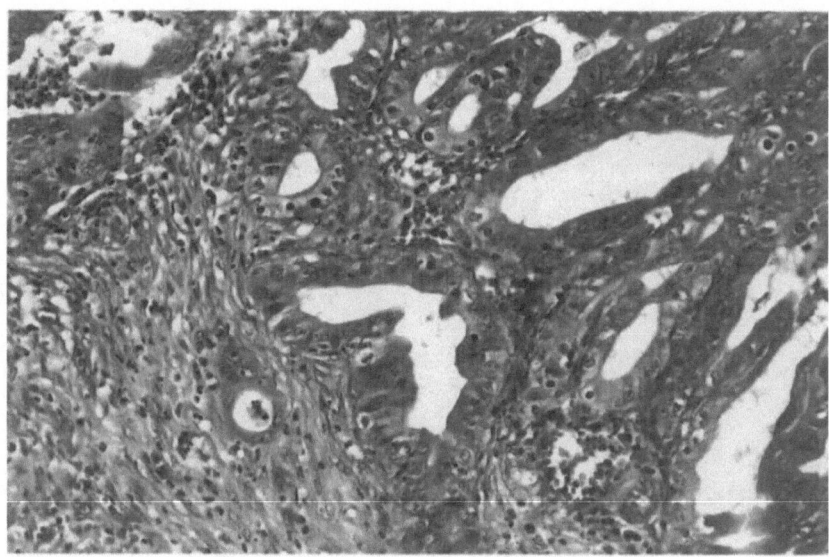

Fig. 33. *Mucinous cystadenocarcinoma, invasive.* The wall of the cystic tumour shows invasive neoplastic glands with poor differentiation

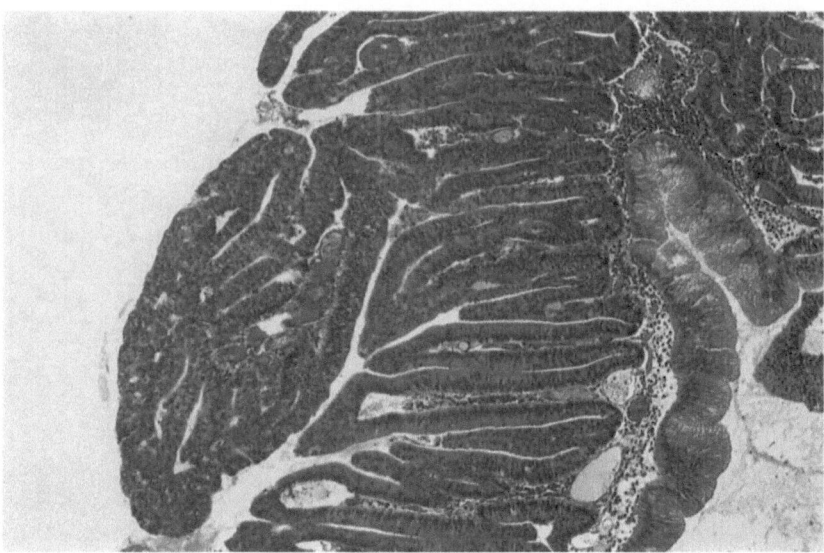

Fig. 34. *Intraductal papillary-mucinous carcinoma.* The tumour tissue shows irregular papillary proliferations which are lined by markedly atypical epithelium

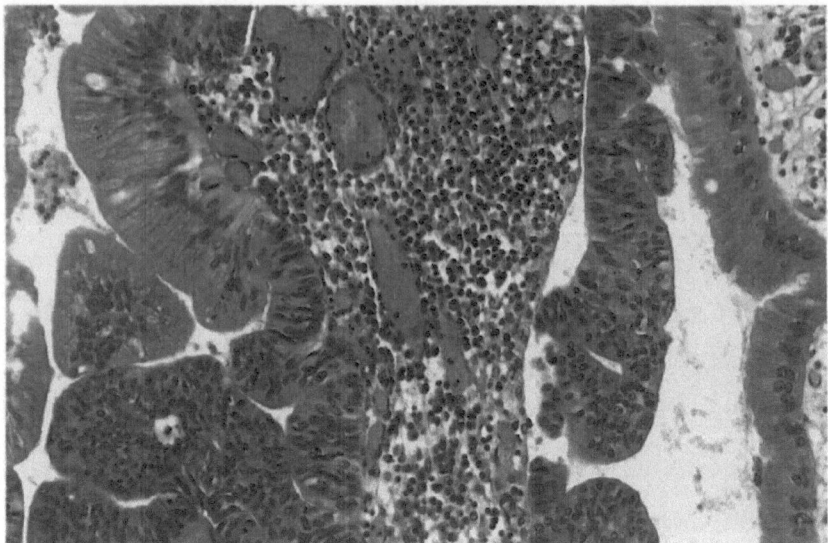

Fig. 35. *Intraductal papillary-mucinous carcinoma, noninvasive.* This high-power view demonstrates severely atypical columnar epithelium adjacent to moderately atypical epithelium

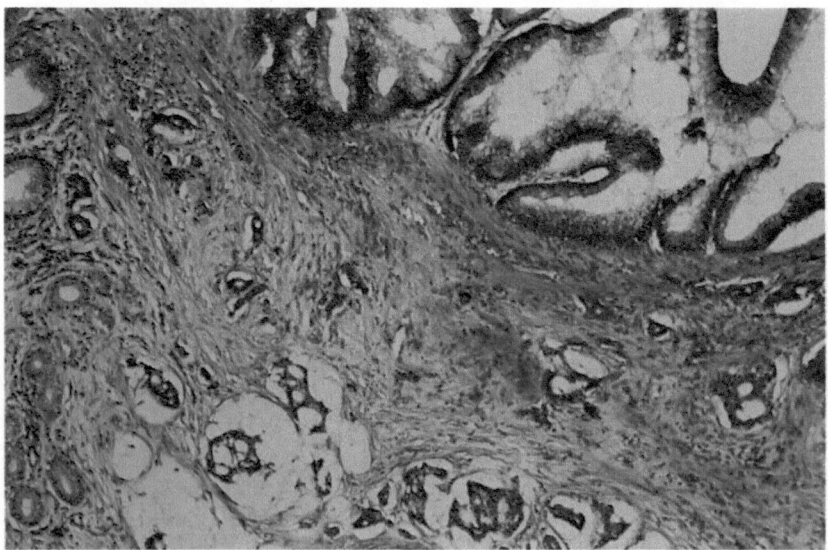

Fig. 36. *Papillary-mucinous carcinoma.* Invasive neoplastic glands with massive mucin production in the pancreatic tissue surrounding a duct involved by intraductal papillary-mucinous carcinoma

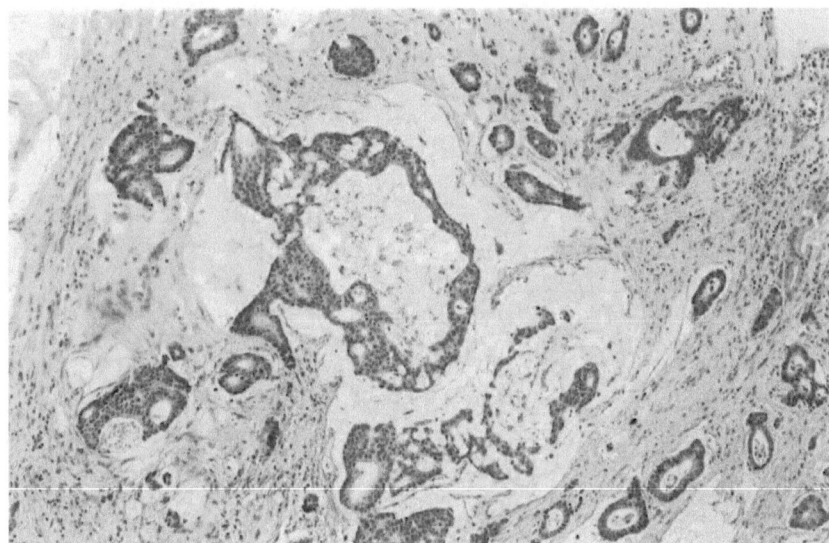

Fig. 37. *Papillary-mucinous carcinoma.* The invasive component of this tumour shows the features of a mucinous noncystic carcinoma

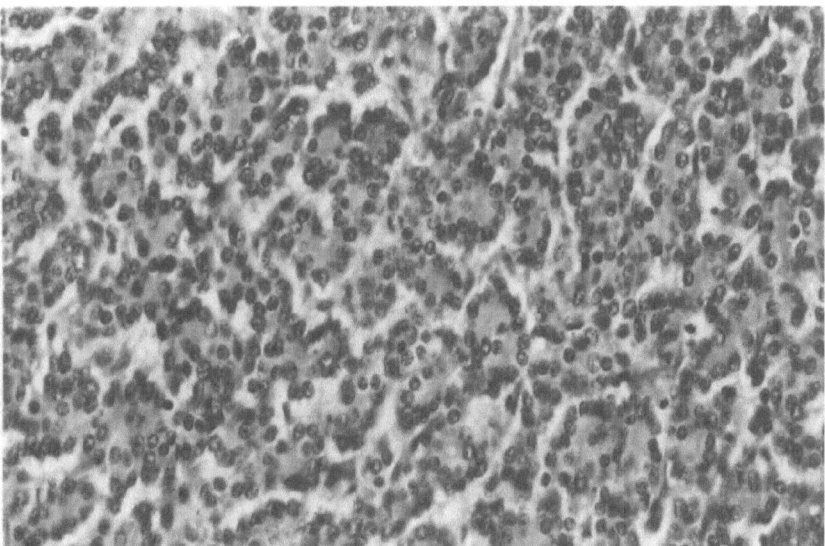

Fig. 38. *Acinar cell carcinoma.* The tissue of this tumour shows a pure acinar pattern, reminiscent of normal pancreatic acinar tissue

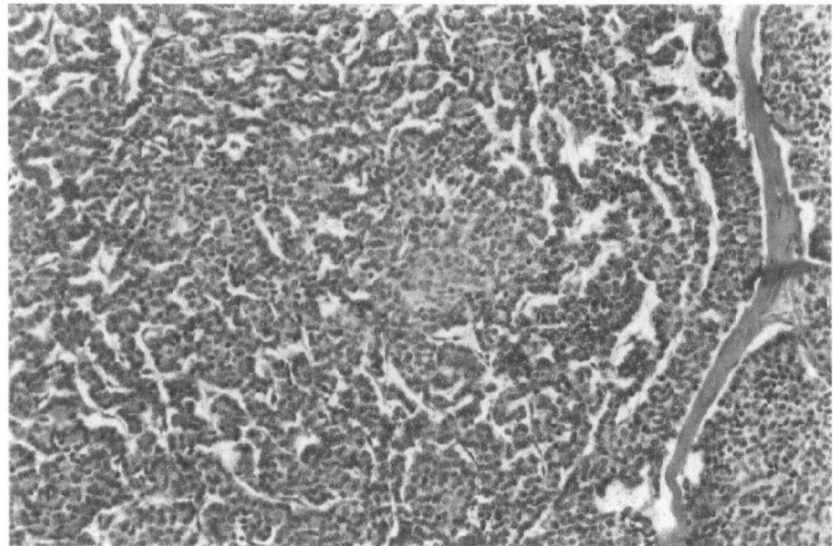

Fig. 39. *Acinar cell carcinoma*. The tissue of this tumour shows a mixed pattern, with acinar areas alternating with trabecular and solid formations. In addition, there is a focus of central necrosis

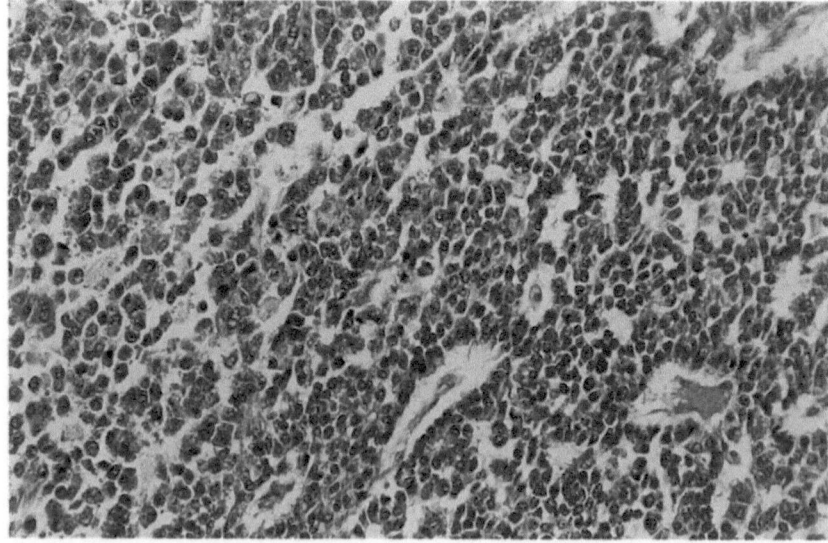

Fig. 40. *Acinar cell carcinoma*. The tissue of this tumour is poorly differentiated and composed of relatively small round cells with scanty cytoplasm

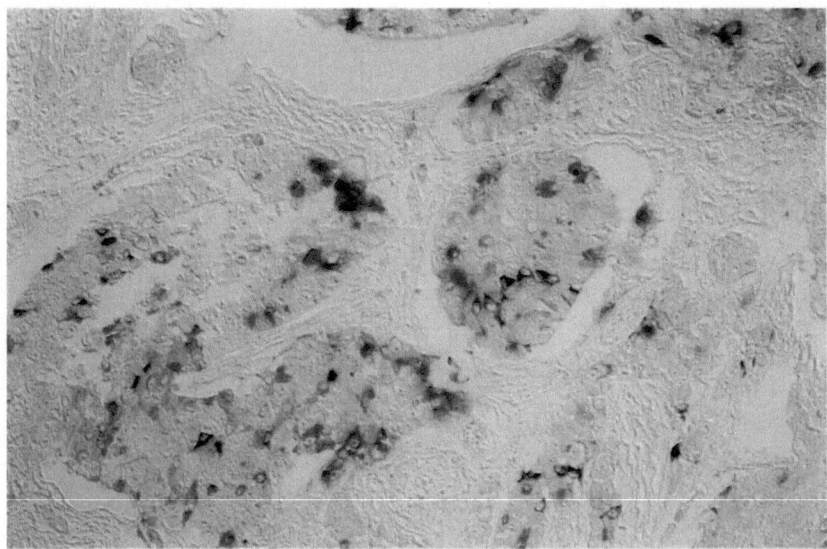

Fig. 41. *Acinar cell carcinoma.* Double immunostaining for trypsin (*blue*) and synaptophysin (*brown*) reveals an admixture of exocrine and endocrine tumour cells

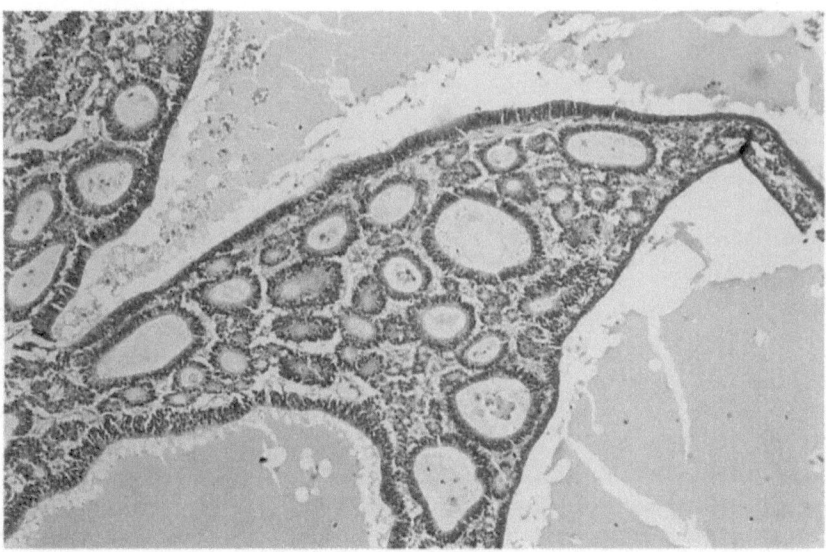

Fig. 42. *Acinar cell cystadenocarinoma.* The tumour tissue shows microcystic structures

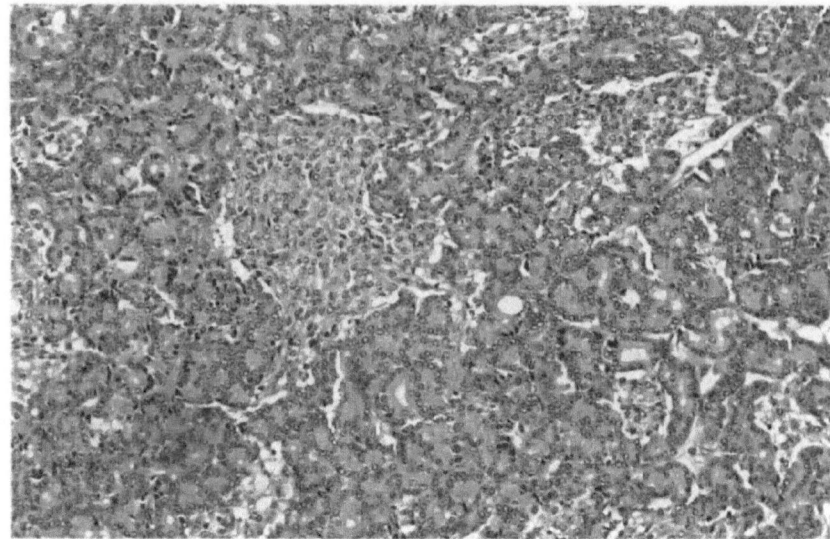

Fig. 43. *Pancreatoblastoma.* The tumour tissue shows an acinar pattern and includes groups of cells with pale cytoplasm (squamoid corpuscles)

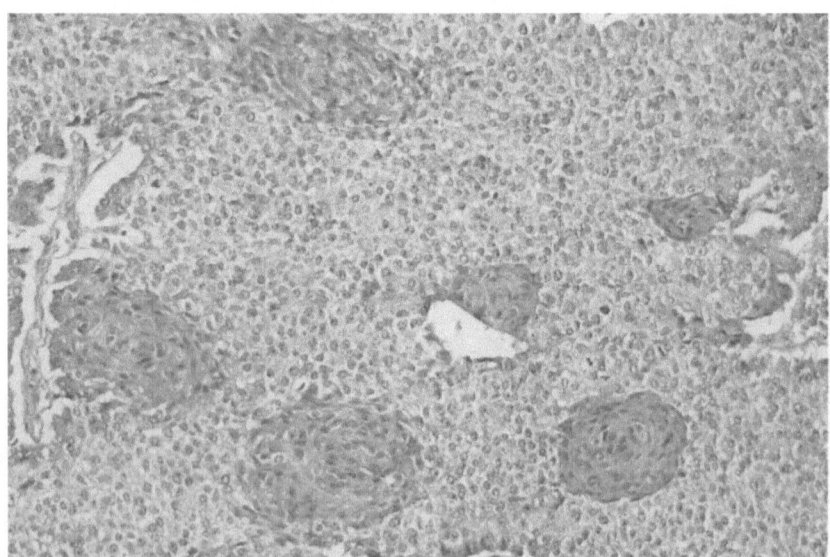

Fig. 44. *Pancreatoblastoma.* Squamoid corpuscles embedded in solid (i.e. undifferentiated) tumour tissue

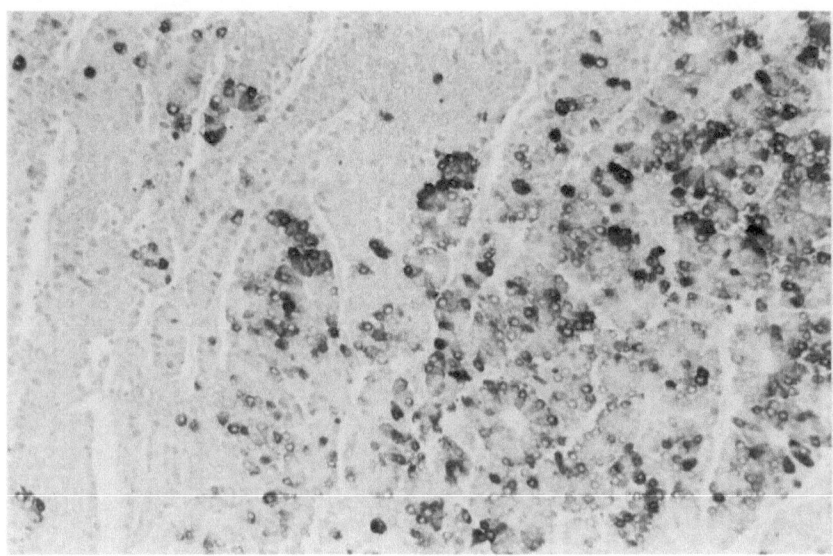

Fig. 45. *Pancreatoblastoma.* Immunostaining for trypsin reveals cytoplasmic positivity in the acinar component of the tumour tissue

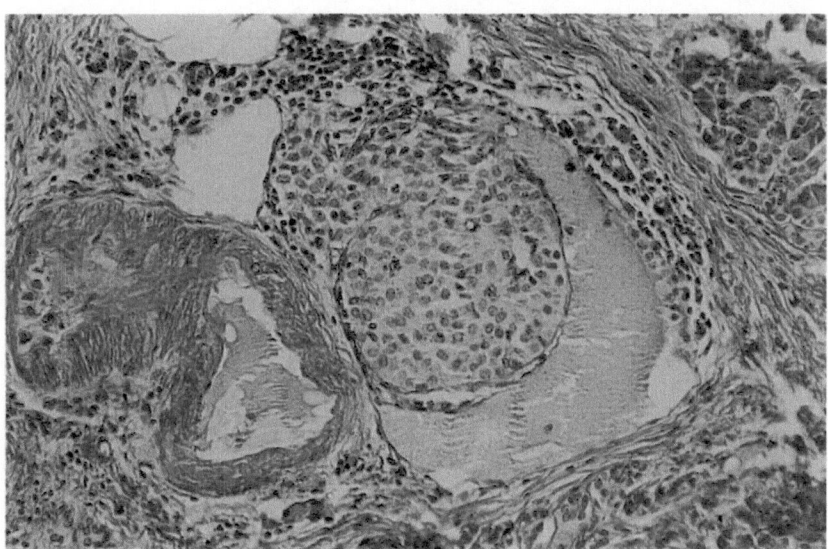

Fig. 46. *Solid-pseudopapillary carcinoma.* Intrapancreatic lymphatic vessel containing tumour tissue

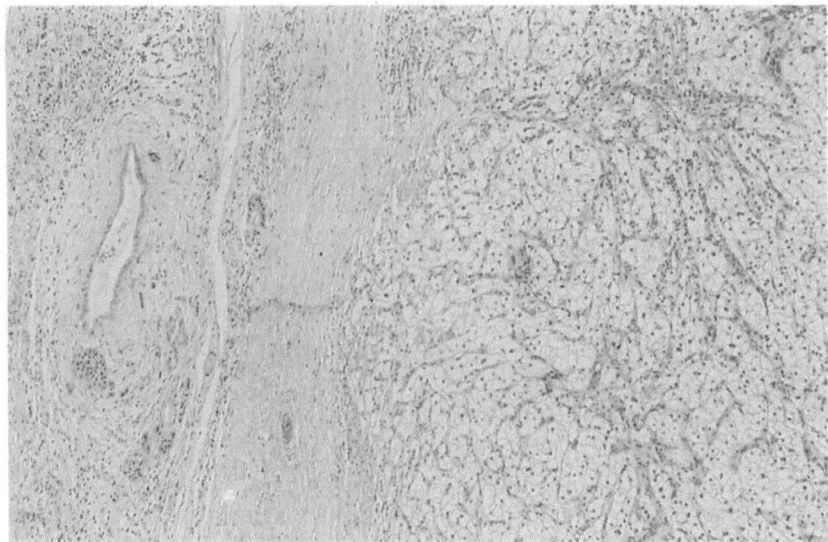

Fig. 47. *Metastasis to the pancreas.* Metastasis of a well-differentiated renal clear cell carcinoma to the pancreas. The tumour tissue is on the *right* and normal pancreatic tissue is on the *left*

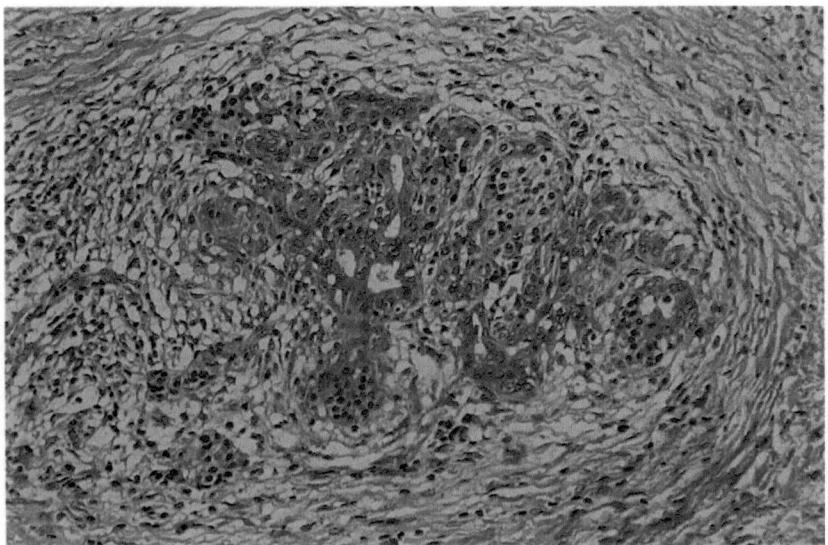

Fig. 48. *Chronic pancreatitis.* Remnant of a pancreatic lobule embedded in sclerotic tissue and infiltrated by inflammatory cells. The residual lobular tissue is composed of small ducts interspersed with endocrine cell clusters

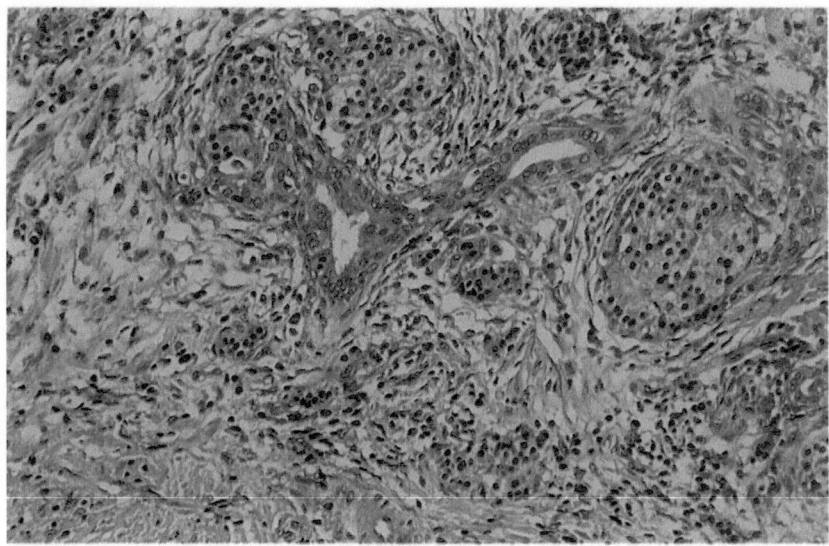

Fig. 49. *Chronic pancreatitis.* Irregularly structured small duct surrounded by islets and loosely arranged connective tissue

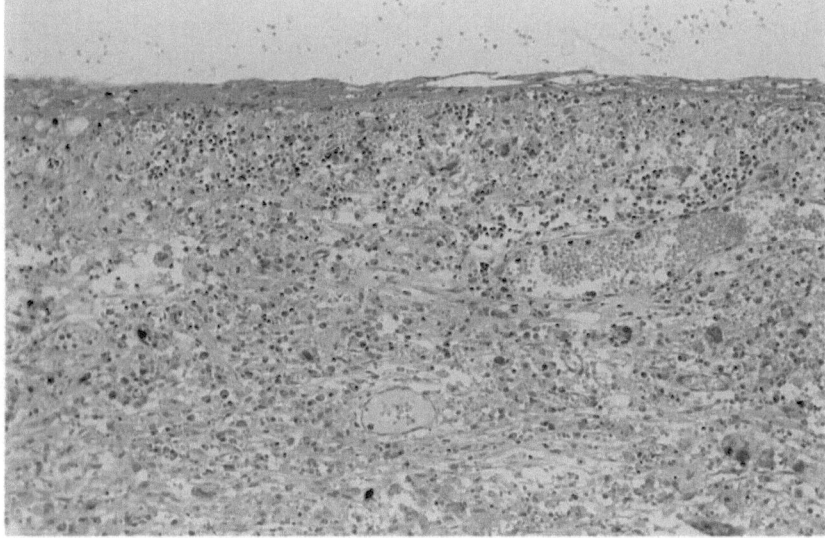

Fig. 50. *Pseudocyst.* Inner layer of the wall of a pseudocyst showing granulation tissue with many macrophages containing hemosiderin pigment

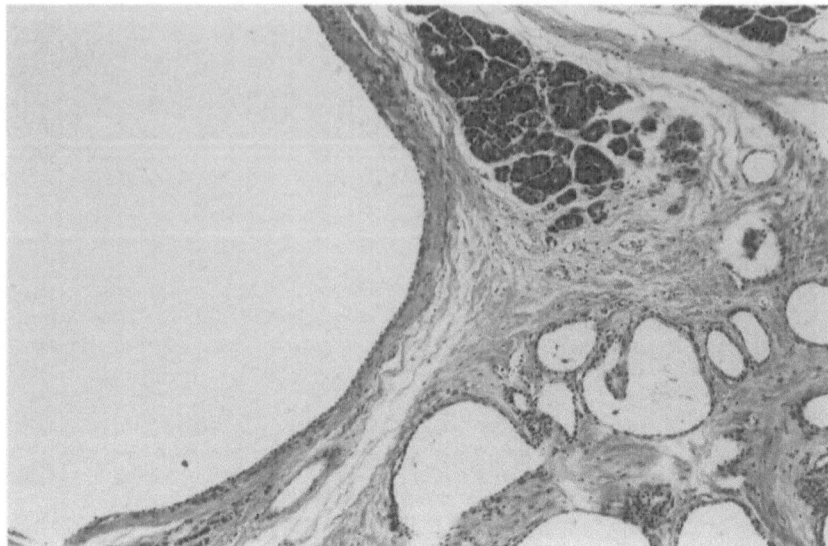

Fig. 51. *Congenital cyst.* The pancreatic tissue of a patient with von Hippel-Lindau syndrome shows small cysts between normal acinar tissue (*upper half*) and normal ducts (*bottom*). The congenital cysts are lined with flattened epithelial cells

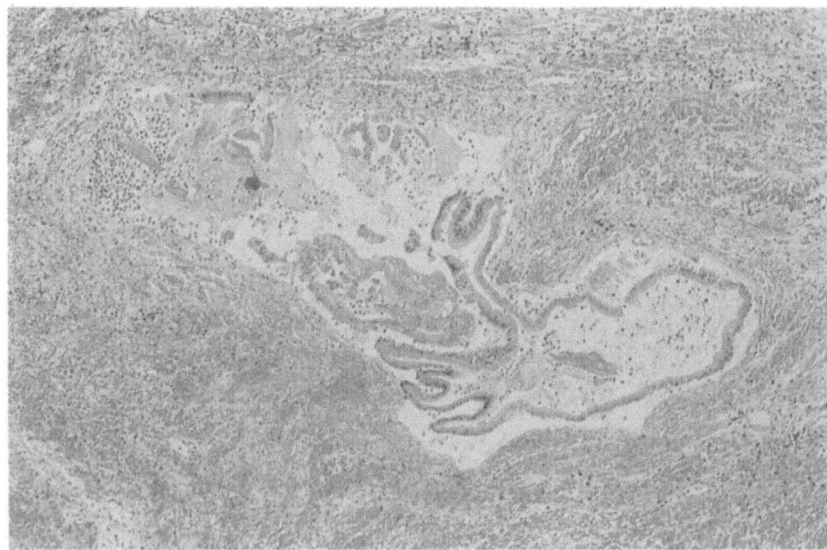

Fig. 52. *Para-ampullary duodenal wall cyst.* The muscular layer of the duodenum contains cysts which are inflamed and partly ruptured. The inflammation spreads into the surrounding tissue

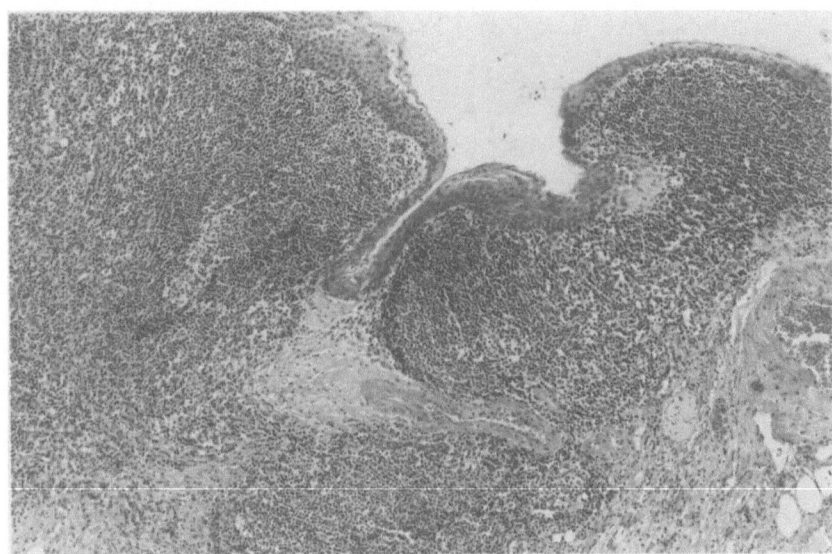

Fig. 53. *Lymphoepithelial cyst.* The wall of the cyst is composed of squamous epithelium which is supported by lymphoid tissue

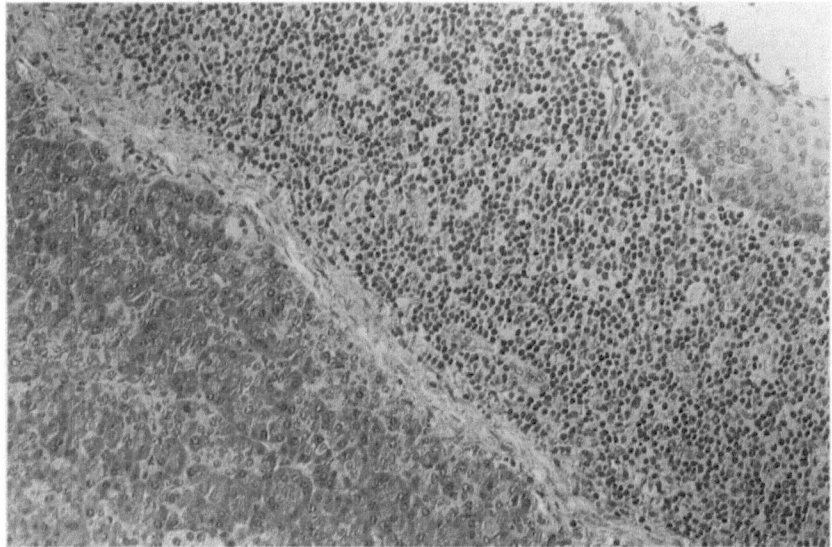

Fig. 54. *Lymphoepithelial cyst.* The squamous epithelium which lines the cyst (*upper right corner*) is separated from the pancreatic tissue (*lower left corner*) by mature lymphoid cells

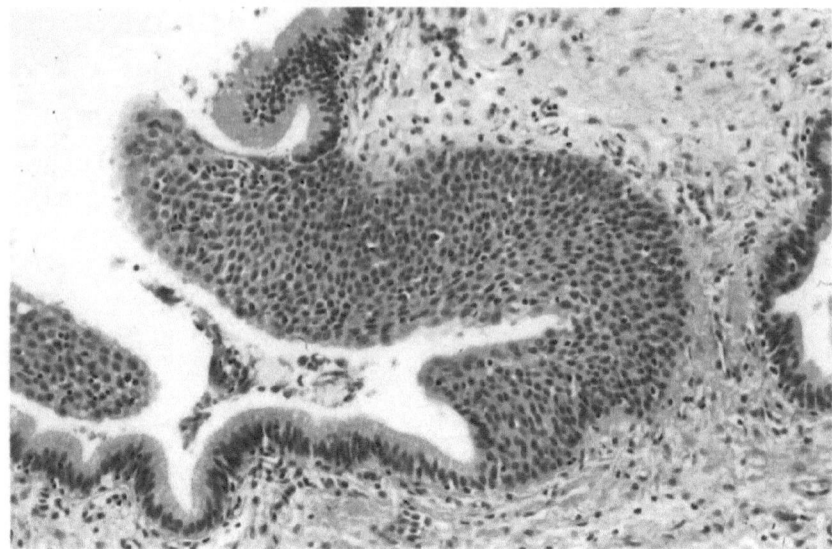

Fig. 55. *Squamous metaplasia.* The main pancreatic duct which carried a catheter is lined by mature squamoid epithelium. The wall of the duct contains mucinous glands

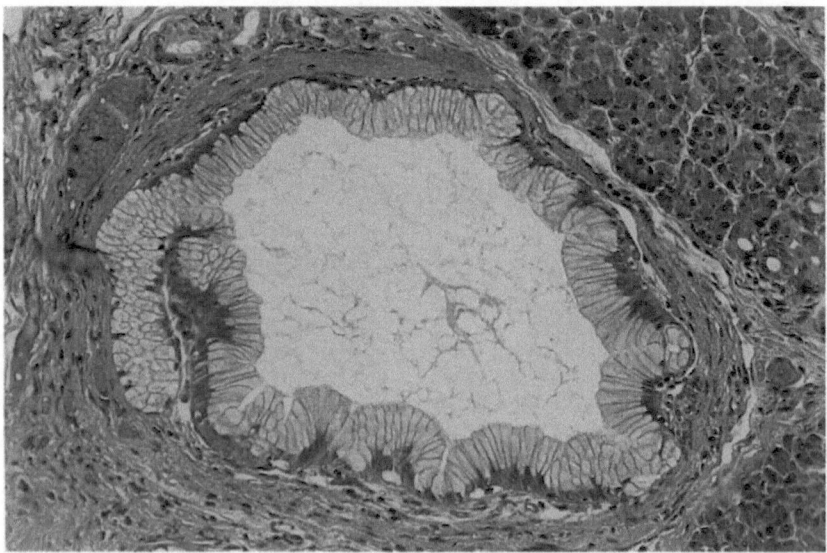

Fig. 56. *Mucinous cell hypertrophy.* The medium-sized duct is lined by large cuboidal cells which show mucin accumulation within the apical cytoplasm

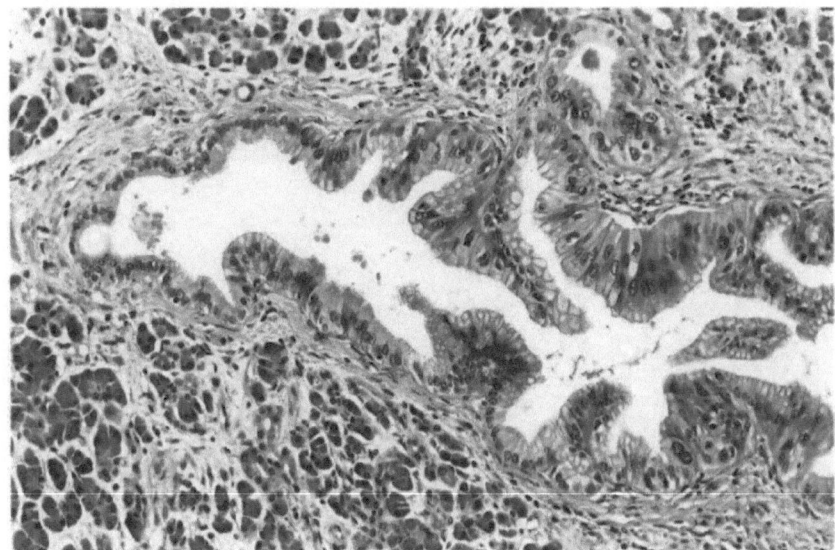

Fig. 57. *Ductal papillary hyperplasia.* Part of a duct showing papillary infolding of the epithelium. The papillary folds are supported by a fibrovascular stalk

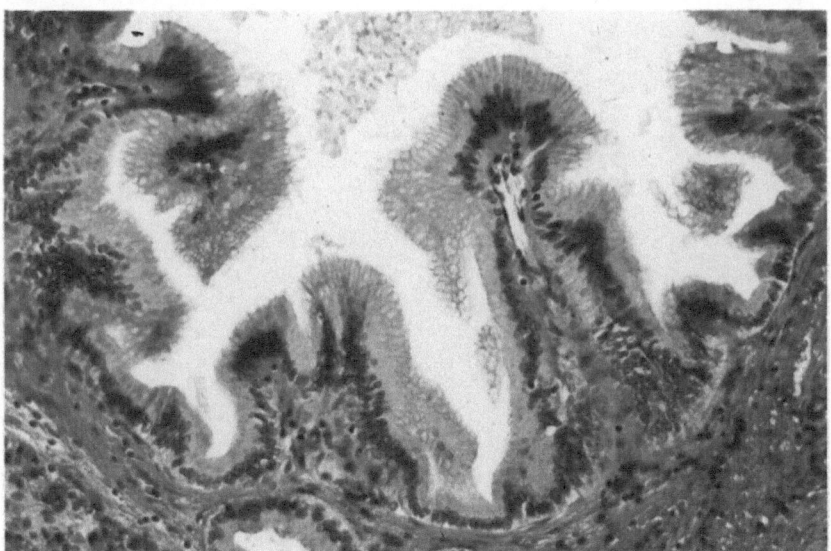

Fig. 58. *Ductal papillary hyperplasia.* The duct epithelium shows mucinous cell hypertrophy. The pseudostratification of the epithelium and the slightly enlarged nuclei suggest mild dysplasia

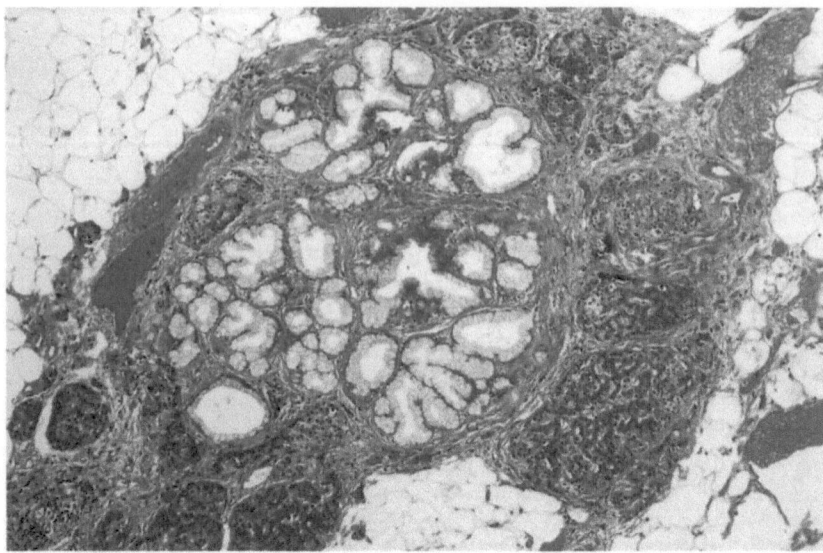

Fig. 59. *Adenomatoid ductal hyperplasia.* The focal lesion consists of an aggregation of small- to medium-sized ducts. The epithelium of the ducts shows mucinous cell hypertrophy

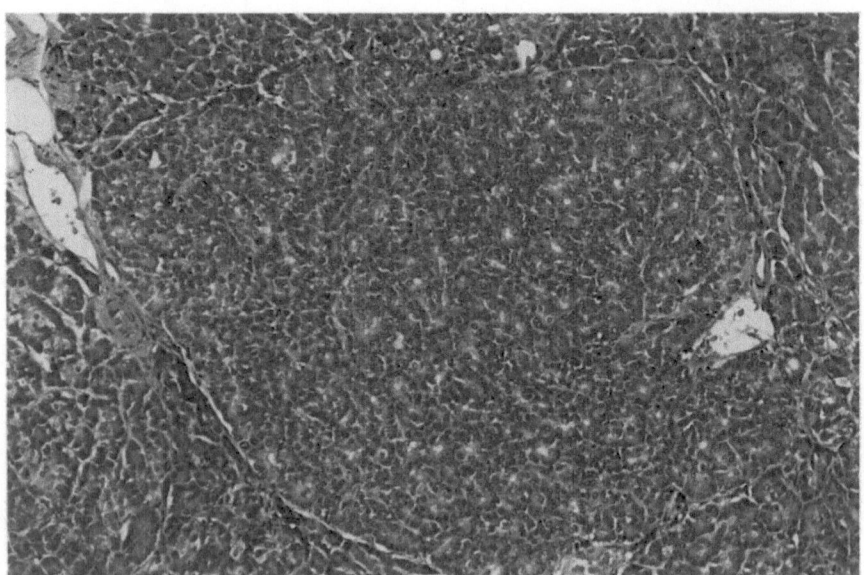

Fig. 60. *Focal acinar cell transformation.* The sharply outlined group of acinar cells shows homogeneous cytoplasmic eosinophilia and slightly reduced nuclear basophilia

Subject Index

Springer
and the
environment

At Springer we firmly believe that an international science publisher has a special obligation to the environment, and our corporate policies consistently reflect this conviction.

We also expect our business partners – paper mills, printers, packaging manufacturers, etc. – to commit themselves to using materials and production processes that do not harm the environment. The paper in this book is made from low- or no-chlorine pulp and is acid free, in conformance with international standards for paper permanency.

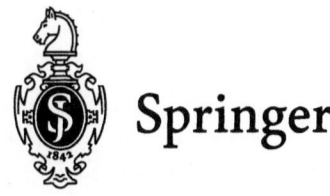

Springer

WHO – International Histological Classification of Tumours

Editor: L. H. Sobin

Chr. Hedinger
Histological Typing of Thyroid Tumours
2nd edition 1988. XII, 66 pages.
92 figures in colour.
Softcover DM 102,–; US $62.00
ISBN 3-540-19244-1

J. R. Jass, L. H. Sobin
Histological Typing of Intestinal Tumours
2nd edition 1989. XII, 126 pages.
136 figures, 8 in colour.
Softcover DM 120,–; US $74.00
ISBN 3-540-50711-6

H. Watanabe, J. R. Jass, L. H. Sobin
Histological Typing of Oesophageal and Gastric Tumours
2nd edition 1990. XII, 108 pages.
120 figures, 8 in colour.
Softcover DM 82,–; US $55.00
ISBN 3-540-51629-8

J. Albores-Saavedra,
D. E. Henson, L. H. Sobin
Histological Typing of Tumours of the Gallbladder and Extrahepatic Bile Ducts
2nd edition 1991. XI, 75 pages.
80 figures, 10 in colour.
Softcover DM 80,–; US $54.95
ISBN 3-540-52838-5

K. Shanmugaratnam
Histological Typing of Tumours of the Upper Respiratory Tract and Ear
2nd edition 1991. XI, 200 pages.
200 figures in colour.
Softcover DM 116,–; US $79.50
ISBN 3-540-53880-1

G. Seifert
Histological Typing of Salivary Gland Tumours
2nd edition 1991. XI, 112 pages.
124 figures in colour.
Softcover DM 76,–; US $59.95
ISBN 3-540-54031-8

I. R. H. Kramer, J. J. Pindborg, M. Shear
Histological Typing of Odontogenic Tumours
2nd edition 1992. XI, 118 pages.
142 figures, 116 in colour.
Softcover DM 75,–; US $59,95
ISBN 3-540-54142-X

P. Kleihues, P. C. Burger, B. W. Scheithauer
Histological Typing of Tumours of the Central Nervous System
2nd edition 1993. XIV, 112 pages.
106 figures in colour.
Softcover DM 144,–; US $89.50
ISBN 3-540-56971-5

■ ■ ■ ■ ■ ■ ■ ■ ■ ■ ■

Please order from
Springer-Verlag Berlin
Fax: + 49 / 30 / 8 27 87- 301
e-mail: orders@springer.de
or through your bookseller

Prices subject to change without notice.
In EU countries the local VAT is effective.

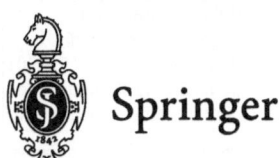

Springer

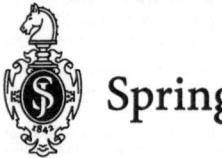